AT RISK

GLOBALIZATION
IN EVERYDAY LIFE

At Risk

Indian Sexual Politics and the Global AIDS Crisis

GOWRI VIJAYAKUMAR

STANFORD UNIVERSITY PRESS
Stanford, California

STANFORD UNIVERSITY PRESS
Stanford, California

Printed in the United States of America on acid-free, archival-quality paper

Library of Congress Cataloging-in-Publication Data
Names: Vijayakumar, Gowri, author.
Title: At risk : Indian sexual politics and the global AIDS crisis / Gowri Vijayakumar.
Other titles: Globalization in everyday life.
Description: Stanford, California : Stanford University Press, 2021. | Series: Globalization in everyday life | Includes bibliographical references and index.
Identifiers: LCCN 2020050233 (print) | LCCN 2020050234 (ebook) | ISBN 9781503627529 (cloth) | ISBN 9781503628052 (paperback) | ISBN 9781503628069 (epub)
Subjects: LCSH: AIDS (Disease)—India—Prevention. | AIDS (Disease)—Political aspects—India. | AIDS (Disease)—Government policy—India. | Sex—Political aspects—India. | Sex workers—Political activity—India. | Sexual minorities—Political activity—India.
Classification: LCC RA643.86.I4 V55 2021 (print) | LCC RA643.86.I4 (ebook) | DDC 362.19697/9200954—dc23
LC record available at https://lccn.loc.gov/2020050233
LC ebook record available at https://lccn.loc.gov/2020050234

Cover design: Christian Storm

Cover photograph: Bangalore, India. Kiran Ln, EyeEm | Alamy

Typeset by Kevin Barrett Kane in 10/14.4 Minion Pro

Contents

Preface

When I tell people this book is about AIDS[1] politics in India, they are often surprised. "Is AIDS still a problem?" they ask. "Is there AIDS in India?" In the US, when AIDS is not a relic of an (assumed white) queer past,[2] it's usually the specter of Africa, not India, that animates the popular imaginary. But the scenario looked different in the mid-2000s, when I first began to learn about AIDS. In 2005, UNAIDS, a joint venture on HIV by eleven United Nations system organizations, estimated that India had the largest AIDS epidemic in the world, with 5.7 million people living with AIDS.[3] Warnings that India's AIDS epidemic would follow the path of sub-Saharan Africa's made global headlines. North American experts predicted that India was on the brink of an explosive crisis and warned that its government, and what they considered a sexually conservative society, were woefully unprepared to stop it. In the next decade, massive resources would be mobilized for the Indian AIDS response.

Around that time, in the summer of 2004, I was an intern with a reproductive health research organization in Durban, South Africa. I had just turned twenty, and I was endlessly curious. It had been ten years since the end of apartheid, and conversations about race, politics, and inequality surrounded me. I had gone to Durban hoping to learn about women's health in the context of a devastating AIDS epidemic. South Africa had (and has)[4] one of the worst AIDS epidemics in the world. Some 5.3 million South Africans were living with HIV in 2004. In KwaZulu-Natal, 37.5% of pregnant women were estimated to be HIV-positive.[5] That summer, I read an article about how the city of Durban had begun to recycle its graves.[6]

As I spent time in Durban, I began to understand the social and political drivers of South Africa's AIDS crisis. I learned about the history of racist population control programs that prioritized reducing Black women's birth rates over their sexual wellness.[7] I learned about the apartheid migrant labor system that created the conditions for AIDS, and the neoliberal patterns of labor exploitation that intensified its effects.[8] I learned about gendered economic precarity and its implications for sexual relationships, power, and control.[9] I saw that AIDS was a symptom of globalization, an index of inequality and marginalization that cut to the heart of the thorny links between race, gender, sexuality, and capitalism.[10] It was that summer that made me a sociologist. I wondered if India's imminent crisis would play out the same way.

Eight years later, when I returned to South Africa, I was beginning a project on AIDS, and I got back in touch with my mentor from 2004. I was surprised to learn that India now featured much more prominently in her work, and in a very different way. No longer an example of a lackluster reaction to an unacknowledged growing threat, India's AIDS response had become a model one. AIDS researchers in South Africa were now collaborating with AIDS researchers in India to develop new strategies for HIV prevention. The organization I had interned with was collaborating with a group in Karnataka, a state in South India, to learn about HIV prevention interventions with sex workers. The coincidence was unexpected. What could South Africa, I wondered, have to learn from India about AIDS? Wasn't India's AIDS epidemic, in which HIV prevalence reached barely one half of 1%, dramatically different from South Africa's? Yet experts from India were helping to develop new approaches for HIV prevention in collaboration with South African experts. The South African minister of health, Aaron Motsoaledi, had visited India to learn about the Gates Foundation's Avahan program. A sex worker activist I interviewed said of the visit, "That was the first time he met a sex worker. And we thought, you can meet a South African sex worker right here! You never asked us!"

From the vantage point of South Africa, India's position on the global AIDS map had changed considerably. Over the short span of less than a

decade, global AIDS experts had gone from seeing India's epidemic as a looming catastrophe to an impressive example of prevention that could provide
models for the rest of the world. In particular, India was often cited, in global
AIDS circles, for its targeted HIV prevention programs with sex workers,
sexual minorities, and transgender people.[11] These prevention programs,
which South Africa's health minister had gone to learn about, emphasized
working with communities considered most at risk of HIV. Indian HIV
prevention efforts, these visits suggested, had been a success. The crisis had
been averted. But how had India gone from a country where conversations
about sex were taboo to a place where sex workers met foreign diplomats? To
what extent did the accounts of globe-trotting experts reflect the realities of
the AIDS response? And what had the effects of HIV prevention programs
been on those at its heart, those targeted as high risk? In short, how had crisis
reshaped Indian sexual politics?

This book argues that the response to India's AIDS crisis transformed,
temporarily, the terrain on which sex workers, sexual minorities, and transgender people engaged the state. India's AIDS response unfolded within a
global set of AIDS institutions made up of donors, UN agencies, other governments, research institutions, and international nongovernmental organizations (NGOs). This set of institutions—which together comprise what
this book considers a *field*—placed countries in a hierarchical and temporal
relationship to each other. Within this field, India was *at risk* of becoming
what Africa had already become. In response, the Indian state sought to contain the risk among sex workers, sexual minorities, and transgender people.
But containment had unexpected effects. This book traces how containing
the crisis created hybrid zones and institutions within the state, in which
groups defined as at risk developed new solidarities and modes of citizenship.
At its heart, this book traces the everyday implications of the global AIDS
response. It charts how India's relationship to the AIDS crisis crystallized
tensions about India's place in the world, and it examines how the Indian
state's response affected the lives of those most targeted for HIV prevention.
How did the risk of a global crisis alter the lives of the groups who came to
embody and represent risk?

Lata[12] illustrates one such trajectory. I was just beginning my fieldwork
when I met her. As we sat on a bench at a Kolkata conference center, grateful
for a little bit of shade, she told me about her organizing work. Lata looked

younger than forty, though there were wrinkles around her eyes, as though she'd been squinting into the sun. A year later, I finally asked if I could interview her with a recorder. Lata was born into a family she classified as scheduled caste (SC) or Dalit.[13] She had been married at fourteen, she told me, sitting on a small cot in her friend's house. The family had refused to introduce her to the intended groom until the day of the wedding. When she finally saw the groom, Lata said, she cried. "Was I really weighing my family down so much? If they'd given me work to do, I'd have done it."

"Their culture was great!" she told me sarcastically of her new in-laws. "You always had to be wearing this wide a *kunkuma* [bright red powder] on your forehead, bangles up to here," (she pointed to her elbow) "and the *pallu* [the loose end of the sari] shouldn't slip; you had to pull it together and pin it. Just look at the tradition in their house! But if you looked inside, it was all rotten!" Any time her father-in law washed his hands, he'd wipe his hands on your sari, she said. When you leaned over to serve his food, his eyes would linger. One night, when everyone else was out of town, he had come into her room and demanded to have sex with her. "I've paid the money and I've gotten you married," he said. "You can't say no to any of the eight of us [men living in the house.]" Lata said she didn't know where the anger and strength came from, but she fought him until he gave up and left. When she told her husband about it, he said if the land belonged to the family, it didn't matter who planted the seeds. Once, while the rest of the family was out of town, her brother-in-law attempted to rape her and, as she fought back against him, she fell into a gutter outside her house. She was seven months pregnant and soon miscarried.

A few years later, after finally leaving her in-laws, beginning a second relationship that ended abruptly, and enduring months of physical and emotional abuse from her own family, Lata found her life at a turning point. Now with two children, one only fifteen days old, Lata began to work at a brick factory. She lived in the factory quarters with her children. There, a friend introduced her to her first clients. "I thought, how long can I take care of the kids with twenty rupees? They give five kilograms of rice and oil. How long can I do this for my kids?" She first worked for an acquaintance, who took nearly half of her earnings as commission, until a client gave her enough money to pay the deposit on her own apartment. Eventually she made enough money to put her children through school. It was an uneven path, but she made a life for them. "This occupation (*vṛtti*) is what filled my hands," she said. Her voice hinted at pride and a twinge of redemption as she described holding an elaborate wedding for her daughter in her family's village. She had invited all her family members to the wedding, the same ones who had once chased her out of her village with a three-year-old daughter and an infant, calling her a whore (*sūḷe*). "For all the pain they gave me," she said, "I wanted to give them something back."

Lata's first contact with a sex worker organization came more than a decade after she first began doing sex work. In 2002, she met a field supervisor from an HIV prevention NGO. The NGO was one of a growing number of HIV prevention NGOs in the state of Karnataka: between 2000 and 2004, the number of targeted interventions with at-risk groups run by NGOs more than doubled to thirty,[14] as part of a nationwide effort at HIV prevention, with a particular focus on states with high HIV prevalence.[15] Starting in 2003, Karnataka became a focus state for the Gates Foundation's US$338-million AIDS program in India, the Avahan initiative. At the time, public health surveillance indicated that 14.4% of women in sex work in Karnataka were HIV positive, and the percentage would jump to 21.6% the following year.[16] In Lata's district in 2004, HIV prevalence among all pregnant women was estimated at 2.5%.[17] Lata herself had not heard of AIDS, but from the NGO, she learned about STIs and HIV.[18] She became a peer educator who kept in contact with sex workers, provided them with condoms, and brought them to clinics to get them tested. Lata became well versed in the language of HIV prevention—meetings, trainings, field visits, peer educators, mapping—and began to monitor regularly the sexual behavior of sex workers she contacted. She filled out forms every week documenting the sexual activities of her regular contacts, keeping track of how many partners they had had, how many times they had had protected sex, and how many condoms she had given them. Through detailed documentation, Lata learned to categorize her contacts as FSW (female sex worker) or MSM (men who have sex with men), and describe FSWs as home-based, street-based, or brothel-based. The stacks of forms on which Lata documented her peers' sexual acts, clients, health status, and condom use would be aggregated weekly and monthly across her zone, city, and state, to form an intricate picture of sexual practice as Karnataka fought off the epidemic.

HIV prevention was Lata's first step into organizations and activism. In 2006, she took a second step: she decided to move to a newly forming activist organization. At a time when HIV prevention programs for sex workers in Karnataka were growing rapidly, the Karnataka Sex Workers' Union was one of the only sex worker organizations in Bangalore not implementing a state-level HIV prevention program. Instead, it focused on legal recognition and workers' rights for sex workers. It was the NGO that brought change to her life, Lata said, but it was the Union that taught her she was no less than anyone else, that if she was unified with others, she could achieve something. She began to speak more openly about her life as a sex worker in meetings. As a Union leader, she traveled around the state and around India and marched in protests against police abuse. She helped Union members obtain ration cards, voter identity cards, and loans and leave abusive partners. She participated in protests of coercive AIDS policies and police violence against sex workers, working-class sexual minorities, and transgender people. She built friendships with kothis[19] and transgender women who organized alongside her.

Lata's activism was one part of the evolution of large-scale social movements focused on sexuality all around India. In 2009, in response to a 2001 writ petition filed by the Naz Foundation, an NGO working on HIV prevention and treatment, the Delhi High Court declared Section 377 of the Indian Penal Code, which criminalized "carnal intercourse against the order of nature," unconstitutional. The case mobilized arguments about the barriers Section 377 posed to HIV prevention, and the National AIDS Control Organization (NACO) filed an affidavit in support of the petition. In 2006, when the Ministry of Women and Child Development introduced a bill in Parliament that proposed amendments to the Immoral Traffic Prevention Act (ITPA), including making paying for sex a punishable crime as a way of curbing sex trafficking, sex worker groups like Lata's across the country protested, with support from NACO, and the bill eventually lapsed in 2009. Lata herself traveled to Delhi to protest the bill. These were national-level shifts, but there were local ones too. In Karnataka in 2005, the director general and inspector general of police issued a circular instructing police officers not to arrest sex workers under ITPA, as a way of reducing the "harassment of the women sex workers." Perhaps most significant were shifts in everyday practices of policing sex work. Lata and other sex worker activists argued case after case in local police stations in which sex workers had been unlawfully detained or assaulted by police. These struggles were about much more than

HIV, but they coincided with, and were partly catalyzed by, the epidemic response.

By the time I met her, Lata was completely different from the young girl married into an abusive family at the age of fourteen. Years later, she bumped into her former husband one day on the way to visit her daughter. "He had forgotten me," she said. "I said . . . you forgot me already? He said I forgot you. Have you seen your wife? I asked. He said she left, why do you ask? I said my God, I'll throw my sandal at you! He said I don't even know you; why are you yelling at me?" Lata collapsed into laughter. "I don't know where he went after that!"

India's predicted AIDS crisis never fully materialized on the scale that had been predicted. And yet massive amounts of money were spent to prevent it. Through the efforts of women like Lata, by 2011, the Karnataka government said over seventy-eight thousand sex workers had been reached with HIV prevention programs.[20] The UNAIDS 2010 *Global Report* noted that "the Indian state of Karnataka has shown evidence that intensive HIV prevention efforts among female sex workers can be highly effective."[21] An article in *The Lancet* found that the Gates Foundation's program, out of its six focus states, was most effective in Karnataka, where it was associated with a 12.7% decline in HIV prevalence.[22] Karnataka's efforts were part of India's global success. One NACO official told me:

UNAIDS . . . look[s] completely to India as a success story. Even on the world stage. If they want to show success, India is one of the countries they always show. We are achieving MDG 6,[23] halting and reversing the epidemic, which means you have to reduce new infections by 50%. India already reduced [new infections] by 56%. In 2015 when we go to the world stage, India will be in the list of countries which have achieved MDG 6. Not many have done it. It's a great example, a silver lining in the dark cloud we have in this country, when we have so many failures, at least something we can show as a success. And they also understand [that], in a country like India, it's difficult to make anything succeed.

This pride in India's success points to how the AIDS crisis was fundamentally tied to ideas about the kind of nation-state India was and could be. In the response to a crisis, states are compared to each other. They become exemplary of certain dynamics, problems, or solutions in a global field, based on, in the case of AIDS, the size of their epidemics, the populations most affected, and the success of their response efforts. The AIDS epidemics in India and sub-Saharan Africa, as my own entry into this book indicates, were defined, understood, and managed in relation to each other. Even though India's predicted AIDS crisis never fully arrived, it carried with it new engagements with global institutions, a new way of thinking about how the Indian state managed sexuality, and new openings for social movements to navigate.

Several months after our interview, Lata left behind activism. Two years later, when I called to tell her I was in town, she told me she had opened a bangle stall. Apart from the fact that Lata's shop was often visited by sex workers who worked in the bus stand and its surrounding area, no one would know from a casual conversation that Lata had spent eight years working in HIV prevention programs, that she had traveled to Kolkata and Delhi to protest the criminalization of sex work. "They came and did something and then they left," she told me. "We still have to be here. They brought us out into the open and then they left us." The AIDS response had temporarily placed Lata at the center of an impending crisis. It had made sex work the defining feature of her winding path through various forms of sexual exchange and violence. Lata had once organized protests on the steps of Town Hall, held meetings with government officials, and given statements to the newspapers. She now lived in the purported aftermath of the crisis. The donors had gone home, the state had moved on, and she was still here. She had returned to the tangle of commerce, intimacy, and survival that had always shaped her life.

When I last visited Lata, in 2019, she was running a flower stall. Every morning she would quickly tie flowers together into elaborate garlands for sale. She was in touch with many friends who did sex work. Though she was no longer involved in HIV prevention work or activism, her friends from her activist and NGO days would visit her with news and gossip every once in a while. By then, Lata was clear she did not want any part in activism. As I sipped juice in a corner of her stall, we talked in code about the work she had done before and the people she had worked with, a time she still vividly remembered. "They brought us out into the open," she said again, when we began talking about the AIDS response. "That time was different. Now, here, in this situation, for this life, I can't be open like I was then." Lata, like many I discuss in this book, was not HIV-positive. But HIV, as the basis for funding, organizational resources, and political access, had temporarily transformed her life.

Today, there are an estimated 2.1 million people living with HIV in India.[24] As AIDS initiatives fade, they have been increasingly forgotten. But the focus of this book is the political implications of AIDS not on those who are living with the virus but on those who, like Lata, live at risk of it. Being defined as at risk opened up new, contradictory ways for sex workers, sexual minorities, and transgender people to relate to the state. It set off transformations in which activist organizations were formed and sustained, and it meant sex workers like Lata developed new ways of speaking, living, and relating to one another, sometimes leading to new hierarchies and exclusions. Some of these shifts were lasting, and some were far more precarious.

AT RISK

1 | INTRODUCTION

> Sex is always political. But there are also
> historical periods in which sexuality is more
> sharply contested and more overtly politicized.
> In such periods, the domain of erotic life is, in
> effect, renegotiated.
>
> *Gayle Rubin*

AS I BEGAN TO MAKE MY WAY from a sex worker health clinic in Nairobi to the nearby minibus taxi (*matatu*) stop, a woman in the waiting area asked very politely if she could have a word with me. Grace was small and thin, with a jagged scar across her mouth. Tentatively, but insistently, she told me she was a sex worker and had previously worked at the clinic as an HIV peer educator. Then she had been arrested while doing sex work. When she was finally released from jail, she found herself destitute. She had three children, she said, one only seven months old. She might be dressed well, she pleaded, as though that might have dissuaded me, but she had nothing. Could I find her a spot in the next peer educator training session? She rifled through her handbag until she found a crumpled business card to show me. I was surprised to see the familiar logo of a sex workers' rights and HIV prevention organization based in Karnataka, India.

How did this business card from Karnataka find its way to a sex worker in Nairobi? Answering this question demands an analysis that moves across scales. It requires an understanding of global institutions: agencies including UNAIDS, UNFPA (United Nations Population Fund, the UN sexual and reproductive health agency), the WHO, and the World Bank and donors like USAID (US Agency for International Development) and the Gates Foundation. These global institutions play a defining role in what this book refers to as a global AIDS field. But understanding Grace's request also requires an understanding of how nation-states govern sexuality within the global AIDS field and how social movements respond to and transform that process of governance. Ultimately, nongovernmental organizations (NGOs), community-based organizations (CBOs) and activists formed the heart of HIV prevention efforts. They formed the context in which Grace, a sex worker, might associate me, a visiting Indian American, with a possible clinic job.

This approach, the one I take in this book, differs from the way many social scientists have studied AIDS. A range of social scientists has written about AIDS, showing that the social and political drivers of AIDS are often missed in biomedical interventions.[1] In India, extensive public health literature assesses the successes of AIDS programs.[2] But what I aim to do in this book is place the analytical focus beyond the drivers of the global AIDS crisis and their possible responses, to the political reconfigurations that ensued from it. In this way, this book is in line with scholarship that considers what the AIDS response can tell us about politics.[3]

Critiques of Indian AIDS programs form a powerful foundation for this book. For decades, scholars and activists have exposed the limits of the response to AIDS in India, arguing that it criminalized and isolated the vulnerable, imposed reified biomedical categories on diverse forms of sexual life, and laid the groundwork for further biomedical intervention.[4] The response to AIDS was always tied up with global institutions: starting in the 1990s, funds and resources for HIV prevention flooded India from bilateral aid agencies, multilateral institutions, and corporate philanthropists. The response to AIDS in India was a global response; it was driven by global funders, agencies, and researchers with money and influence. This book builds on these critiques by analyzing how global institutions responded to the crisis on the terrain of politics—at the interface of the Indian state and Indian social movements.[5] By the time it closed its doors, even the famous Gates Foundation program in India was forced to recognize the centrality of the state and social movements in addressing AIDS.[6]

This book argues that the global AIDS crisis temporarily transformed the terrain on which sex workers, sexual minorities, and transgender people[7] engaged the state, both individually and collectively. The global AIDS crisis created a field that positioned nation-states in relation to each other. Within this field, African countries were *in crisis*, and India was *at risk* of one. AIDS experts considered sex workers, sexual minorities, and transgender people to embody the heart of this risk. But these groups were criminalized and stigmatized. To respond, state officials created hybrid institutions within the state that were insulated from the rest of a slow-moving and sexually conservative bureaucracy and intimately linked to global networks of experts and activists. Within these spaces, state officials could engage sexuality in new ways to prevent AIDS—moving from tactics of criminalization and marginalization to tactics of incorporation and inclusion. These institutional openings allowed state officials to contain risk, while creating hybrid sites within which sex workers, sexual minorities, and transgender people could experiment with new ways of articulating sexual identity and develop new strategies for engaging the state.

Social scientists have written about risk as an increasingly powerful organizing logic for politics. As the "anticipation of catastrophe," risk creates a "global community of threats,"[8] ranging from terrorism to economic collapse. But, as this book shows, risk is defined in relation to race, gender, sexuality, and geopolitics. In the case of AIDS, being marked *at risk* both built on and reinforced existing relations of hierarchy and exclusion.[9] In order to contain the risk of becoming *like Africa*, India had to contain the groups that presented an internal threat to the nation's morality, its gendered and sexual *others*.

The AIDS crisis was an opening into the remaking of Indian sexual politics, then, because it cut to the heart of tensions about the kind of nation-state India was and could be. Within the global AIDS field, AIDS epidemics and responses were compared, measured, and developed in relation to each other. For state officials, how India governed AIDS indexed India's emergence as a modern, technically advanced nation-state that could respond to crisis with pragmatism and foresight. In extending its analysis to Kenya, this book charts how, throughout the AIDS response, the Indian state, and Indian sexuality, came to be represented, within this global AIDS field, as an alternative path to the devastation in sub-Saharan Africa. At the small clinic for Nairobi's sex workers where Grace sought employment, several HIV experts from India had arrived in the last two years to conduct training and research. In this context, Grace could be forgiven for confusing me with other notebook-wielding middle-class Indian women who had passed through the clinic. The travel of HIV prevention strategies from India to Kenya reflected global institutions' efforts to compare and categorize nation-states. But this process inadvertently opened up possibilities for redefining what sexuality meant, within India and also beyond it.

INDIA AT RISK AND THE GLOBAL AIDS CRISIS

How did India come to be understood as at risk of an AIDS crisis? One important starting point is the disproportionate global funding for AIDS in the mid-2000s. Early commentators, writing from India, warned that the AIDS crisis was mostly the exaggerated invention of Western experts and global agencies,[10] foreshadowing later charges of AIDS exceptionalism.[11] Some of this wariness is reflected in the numbers. Recent estimates suggest that about 0.22% of Indian adults are living with HIV; this figure has never gone above 0.5%.[12] Yet in 1999, donors committed US$275 million to AIDS and STD programs in India, more than they did for the rest of the health sector combined.[13] This response seems outsized even when taking into account the fact that India's large population means that it is home to 2.1 million people living with HIV, giving it the third-largest HIV epidemic in the world.[14] Researchers from the Million Death Study in the early 2000s estimated that 120,000 adults in India (ages 15–69) died of malaria per year[15] and about 100,000 (ages 15–59) from AIDS-related causes.[16] But in 2006, donors disbursed $19 million of official development aid for malaria control in India, compared to $108 million for AIDS and STDs.[17] AIDS exceptionalism is a global pattern. In 2007 globally, nearly the same amount of official development assistance was committed to STD and AIDS control and the health sector—$7.8 billion and $7.6 billion respectively.[18] While this funding distribution began to shift slightly after the mid-2000s, funding for AIDS remains relatively significant.[19] UNAIDS reports that, accounting for all funding sources, $18.6 billion was available for AIDS programs at the end of 2019.[20]

This exceptional response suggests that what constitutes a crisis has never been a straightforward matter of quantity or scale. Instead, crises are defined and responded to within a global field, shaped by global institutions.[21] Global institutions place states within a hierarchical order that determines which states are most effective and which most irresponsible. These judgments are moral as well as technical.[22] The Indian state did not respond to AIDS primarily because it recognized it as an immediate public health challenge: other major infectious diseases, like malaria and tuberculosis, let alone basic public health and sanitation, compete for its attention with less success. Instead, the Indian state responded primarily because of the pressure to manage the risk of crisis—risk that was defined within this global field.[23]

A field, for the sociologist Pierre Bourdieu, consists of "a network, or a configuration, of objective relations between positions."[24] In simpler terms, in the context of AIDS, a field is made up of the institutions and people who are affected by, or involved in, managing the disease, and see themselves as participating in a shared set of relationships and conversations about how to respond. Within this field, different institutions and actors struggle for status and resources. There are particular rules to the game. There are also hierarchies in which some actors are subordinate and some are dominant. The anthropologist and activist akshay khanna notes that the HIV industry forms its own linguistic community: "Those who work on HIV . . . speak a particular language, engage in particular practices, are organized in particular ways and circulate within a closed circle in terms of jobs."[25] Though fields can overlap with other fields, khanna suggests that they have a distinct internal logic and order of relationships. Not everyone in a field takes the same position or believes the same things, but when debates emerge or conflicts take hold, the members of a field are speaking to one another.[26]

Bourdieu saw fields mainly within the boundaries of the nation-state. But fields can also be understood globally, as relationships among nation-states shaped and structured by global institutions that often set the rules.[27] In the context of a global crisis, nation-states' navigation of global fields becomes particularly urgent. The AIDS crisis evoked ideas of a global moral community with the responsibility to respond, and nation-states were held to account within this moral community for their action or inaction. Statistics and epidemiological data played a key role in this comparison and ranking;[28] they served to "summarize, reassemble, simplify and rank" states in terms of their AIDS epidemics.[29] The crisis created openings for intervention, for the linking of everyday life to global geopolitics, and for the exercise of massive institutional resources in unlikely places. It demanded that states adopt unusual practices and generate exceptional spaces. This made AIDS an unlikely but potent political force.

AT-RISK GROUPS AND INDIAN SEXUAL POLITICS

In situating the AIDS crisis within Indian sexual politics, this book builds on the insight that ideas of sexuality are, as Patricia Hill Collins puts it, the "fulcrum" for constructing difference around race, caste, gender, and class, and are thus fundamental to power relations.[30] In accounts of global institutions and global fields, scholars have often overlooked the role of gender and sexuality in mediating states' relationships to them. But feminist and queer scholars have long shown us that gender and sexuality are, in fact, crucial to how global politics operate.[31] This scholarship suggests that sexuality is central both to what states do—how they govern sexuality— and what they represent nationally and globally. On the one hand, the state manages, regulates, and shapes sexuality within the nation. On the other, the idea of the state itself is upheld through sexual and gendered imaginaries.[32] These two enterprises often find themselves at odds. The business of regulating sexuality is often contradictory and uneven, while, at the same time, states project an idea of unity, a *state effect*[33] that can take on its own political life. The management of sexuality and gender helps to sustain this state effect.[34] In the global field, ideas of sexual desirability, tolerance, and progress help to distinguish nation-states from each other as they compete for political and economic capital.[35] States, particularly those in the global South, are often pushed to answer for their progress on issues of gender, and increasingly sexuality, within global humanitarian fields.

AIDS suggests a particularly potent moment in which the capacities of states were contested and renegotiated. The global crisis crystallized tensions about what kind of nation-state India was. Was it modern or backward, effective or incompetent? The fact that AIDS was a sexual crisis tied these questions to fundamental concerns about Indian sexuality on the global stage. The AIDS crisis carried with it concerns and debates about India's moral and sexual character. It laid bare the meanings of Indian sexuality at a time when India was becoming a rising geopolitical power. Thus, India's engagement with the global AIDS field at the moment of crisis became an opening into renegotiating Indian sexuality. It forced the state to acknowledge the sexual others who embodied risk.

In response to the AIDS crisis, this book shows, the Indian state's regulation of sexuality underwent a decisive shift. Until the 1980s, and up through the early AIDS response, the Indian state continued the repressiveness of colonial legal precedent. M. Jacqui Alexander writes that, in moments of crisis, states are particularly likely to criminalize deviant sexuality, because sexuality is so deeply bound with ideas of the state's authority.[36] In the Indian context, the heterosexuality of the state[37] had long been sustained by isolating and containing those who put it *at risk*—whether during the Contagious Diseases Acts,[38] which subjected women in prostitution to a punitive medical regime, or through the criminalization of sodomy.[39] The early AIDS response tapped into a range of tensions about national belonging that marked Dalits, sex workers, queer people, and (Black) foreigners as a threat.[40] As activists from the AIDS Bhedbhav Virodhi Andolan (ABVA, or Movement Against AIDS-Related Discrimination) at the time powerfully argued, the early AIDS response isolated sex workers and gay men as the carriers of high risk, clinging to an "idea that the 'high-risk activities' associated with HIV transmission take place only on the periphery of a mythically constructed 'general population,'"[41] imagined as elite, dominant-caste, Hindu married women.

This strategy of risk containment persisted as an organizing logic of India's HIV prevention response. A NACO operational guidelines document from 2007 explains the epidemiological logic of its targeted intervention program. "Core high-risk groups (HRGs)," defined as "female sex workers (FSWs)," "high risk men who have sex with men (MSMs)," "transgenders (TGs)," and "injecting drug users (IDUs)," were those who had "higher levels of risk"; transmission beyond this group occurred through "bridge populations," such as clients of sex workers, to the "general population." This pattern made it "most effective and efficient to target prevention toward HRG members."[42] Focusing on these high-risk groups, and containing HIV within them before it could reach the general population, was more effective than attempting large-scale changes in behavior.

But as the Indian state's response to AIDS evolved, this strategy of containing those at risk shifted to a strategy of incorporation. The risk of crisis put pressure on the Indian state to pursue fast, decisive action, exceptional strategies, and temporary suspensions of conventional sexual moralities. It required autonomous administrative structures. UNAIDS formed in 1994 with the mandate of operating across existing UN agencies to respond more efficiently to the epidemic. It also created concentrations of resources in situations of scarcity.[43] These pockets within the state, as Erin McDonnell calls them, could become sites for experimentation.[44]

Indian feminist and queer activists and scholars have sharply criticized the AIDS industry for depoliticizing and bio-medicalizing sexuality and for reproducing caste and class hierarchies.[45] In a particularly powerful Dalit queer critique, for example, Surya writes, "Before HIV funding oiled and co-opted 'queer,' before it recreated and held in place caste hierarchies—Indian collective queer spaces were found in hamams, and bastis, and parks. . . . it's hard to tell from the rainbow flagged, pride marching exuberance, and the Savarna stamp of approval on the HIV prevention project—but the queer movement in India is a Dalitbahujan movement."[46] At the same time, scholars and activists have also noted that HIV prevention programs have created opportunities for social and political mobility and spaces in which activists could redirect resources to their struggles.[47] Akhil Katyal notes that HIV prevention NGOs "have dotted both cities and small towns in India and have become some of the most interesting sites of experiments between idioms, often cutting across class and language."[48] These spaces, Katyal notes, create "further categories and terms that can be made into sites of intervention," but they also enable people to mobilize global terms of political inclusion that can be repurposed. Indeed, a range of Indian feminist and queer scholars have noted the contradictory effects of the AIDS response, which has introduced new forms of surveillance but also, as Nivedita Menon puts it, "opened the floodgates for political articulation of non-normative sexualities"[49] in ways that have reproduced but also sometimes challenged dominant sexual regimes. Many who are not HIV-positive have shaped, and been shaped by, these designations and rearticulations of risk.

This book offers an ethnographic perspective on this fraught interface between global crisis response and sexual politics. I show that HIV drop-in centers did become sites for reproducing forms of gendered respectability reinforced by class and caste, but also that they became sites for contestation, as sex workers, sexual minorities, and transgender people used them to make citizenship claims on the state and negotiate visibility on their own terms. These negotiations point to what feminist and queer scholars have long noted about how states govern gender and sexuality, and the workings of the Indian state in particular. These scholars point to the state as posing complex, fraught possibilities rather than as operating as a singular site of patriarchal control or violence.[50] The state and civil society are contradictory terrains for women and sexual minorities, regulating sexual activity, generating sexual categorizations, and serving as a target of sexual activism all at the same time.[51] Aradhana Sharma points to how the Indian state operates through relationships with NGOs and social movement organizations "whose autonomy from state institutions remains contested and partial."[52] In responding to AIDS, the Indian state served as an unpredictable site of contestation.[53]

Thinking about AIDS as an opening for struggle for sex workers, sexual minorities, and transgender people implies a different way of thinking about states than has long been common for sociologists. Especially in comparative and transnational research, sociologists have often understood the state as a unitary actor. But states rarely operate in a singular way. More recently, sociologists have called for more multifaceted understandings of the state that disaggregate its often conflicting and overlapping components. As Tianna Paschel argues, national activists can exploit fields at different scales, using alignments with global fields and state agencies to advance their cause.[54] There are both "many hands on the state"[55]—as states are positioned in relation to each other within global fields—and "many hands of the state"[56]—as states are multifaceted, internally contradictory, and linked to social movements. Sexual crises offer moments when battles over governance and representation, within and across states, gain heightened urgency. And in the process of responding to crises, activists can articulate the stakes of a crisis in a range of ways. India's predicted AIDS crisis never fully arrived, but it brought with it a global apparatus of funding and discourses that transformed the terrain on which gender and sexuality were articulated, individually and collectively. By tracing these transformations, this book helps to demonstrate how feminist and queer perspectives are essential to the sociology of the state and global institutions.

METHODS AND SITES

In writing about the possibilities for ethnography in a transnational context, Michael Burawoy argues that "the global [is] produced in the local," and that "globalization is the production of (dis)connections that link and of discourses that travel."[57] By following these connections and threads, ethnography can illuminate "the lived experience of globalization."[58] This book attempts to live up to the promise of global ethnography.

The institutions, funding flows, and activist alliances that make up the global AIDS response are dizzyingly complicated. When I returned from my first foray into fieldwork with a scribbled diagram full of curving arrows and multiple organizations, cities, and countries, my graduate advisors quickly urged me to rethink the more traditionally comparative framework with which I had, rather naively, begun. The resulting book focuses on linkages across sites rather than comparisons; I focus, for example, on how AIDS experts redesigned HIV prevention strategies from India in Kenya rather than compare the two countries as though the two AIDS responses were separate and disconnected. In taking this approach, I draw inspiration from a diverse disciplinary lineage. From critical geography, for example, I draw on Jamie Peck and Nik Theodore's provocation to *follow the policy* of AIDS programs across disparate sites that link experiences of the global AIDS field, Gillian Hart's skepticism of top-down "impact models" of globalization, and Doreen Massey's insistence on a "global sense of place" rooted in an understanding of the racial, gendered, and political economic dynamics within particular sites where transnational flows intersect.[59] Drawing on transnational feminist and queer studies, I center colonial and postcolonial transnational power relations across and within sites.[60] Vrushali Patil's concept of "webbed connectivities" or Gurminder Bhambra's "connected sociologies" further illuminate this approach, foregrounding the colonial and imperial histories of transnational linkages, across seemingly disparate formations of race, gender, and sexuality.[61] These scholars push sociologists to think about transnational connections rather than isolated ideal types. Here, I draw on these insights to illuminate connections across disparate institutional sites, political formations, and sexual terrains.

Because this book operates across different scales, studying global institutions, national states, NGOs, CBOs, and social movements, it uses a diverse methodological toolkit. The bulk of the book is based on 153 in-depth interviews, eighteen months of participant observation, and analysis of policy documents and newspaper articles. My in-depth interviews include fifty with AIDS experts at the local, regional, national, and global levels; eighty-two with activists and HIV peer educators in Bangalore, and twenty-one in Nairobi and Mombasa. My participant observation draws on informal participation in meetings, public events, and protests and everyday hanging out in HIV drop-in centers run by community-based organizations. My textual analysis included academic articles; NGO, government, and donor reports; and organizational websites. I used 135 medical journal articles from the years 1985 to 1995 and a subset of about fifty opinion and review articles to map debates over India's AIDS crisis. I also reviewed about fifty newspaper articles in the *Times of India* and the *New York Times*.

My ethnographic fieldwork focuses specifically on the city of Bangalore. Bangalore was a useful site for several reasons. First, Bangalore was one of several home bases for AIDS experts from African countries as well as the US and Canada conducting research and training and linking India to the global AIDS field. Bangalore is the capital of Karnataka, a *high-prevalence* state for AIDS, which made it a focus of global AIDS funding, including from the Gates Foundation.[62] Second, Bangalore was home to organizations with diverse orientations and alliances working on HIV prevention. Third, Bangalore was a place where I spoke the official language, Kannada, and was a city I knew well enough to understand the trajectory of HIV prevention policies within its locally specific political context. My comfort in navigating the city primed me to notice dynamics outside of the AIDS industry.[63] I might have missed these dynamics if my starting point had been the lens of AIDS alone.

A global ethnographic approach requires an openness to research sites. For me this meant a willingness to follow threads my interviewees suggested. I used this approach to follow the policy to Nairobi. I chose Nairobi because the Kenyan government was in the process of revising its approach to HIV prevention based on what officials I interviewed described as "the Indian experience." Observing how Indian HIV prevention programs were represented and adapted in Kenya illuminated how the Indian state was positioned in the global AIDS field, both symbolically, in terms of ideas of India's state capacity, and materially, in terms of its access to funds. It also allowed me to understand how different actors—the state, donors, NGOs, CBOs, and activists—with distinct goals played a role in this positioning. In short, it allowed me to analyze the relationship between struggles over AIDS and sexuality within India and their representation in the global field. Scholarship on gender and sexuality often stops at understanding the relationship between India and the West. Here, by offering a more multidimensional perspective on the place of India's AIDS crisis in relation to both Africa and the West, I open up new ways of understanding how Indian sexuality is understood and regulated, as the Indian state contends with both its internal exclusions and its place in the world order.[64] I also demonstrate how these struggles in the global field can be premised on deep-seated racial hierarchies.

If studying global institutions poses particular methodological challenges, studying states does, too. In the postcolonial Indian bureaucratic context, Weberian delegation of authority often becomes a maze of deflection, where the "real" work of governance always appears to happen "somewhere else." Recent works by Nayanika Mathur and Jyoti Puri both open with striking ethnographic accounts of the researcher navigating bureaucratic offices, repeatedly being told that the object of their research is either far away or nowhere to be found.[65] Shifting the site of research to the interface between the state bureaucracy and social movements can pose a further set of challenges. Tianna Paschel notes, for example, how studying social movements with various divisions can mean the researcher's own loyalties are questioned.[66] Ideological differences, including differences in ways of engaging (or being co-opted by) the state, mean the researcher is often asked to locate oneself on shifting terrain. Over the course of fieldwork, I found my way from activists to state agencies to researchers and funders in what I soon discovered was a tightly-knit space of debate and contestation. Long before I began to order my data into an argument about the fragile interface of state agencies, social movements, and global institutions that made up the Indian AIDS response, the process of fieldwork had already made the vibrancy of those relationships clear.

In navigating the shifting terrain of the AIDS response in the years I studied it, I had to make choices to narrow down the scope of my fieldwork and my argument. The book places a slightly heavier emphasis on the relationship between the AIDS response and the politics of sex work than it does on the politics of homosexuality and queer love; other recent books analyze the latter.[67] It does not address the full range of concerns that shape the AIDS epidemic in India or globally; in focusing on AIDS as a sexual crisis, this book follows the overwhelming focus of Indian and global AIDS programs, funding, and popular discourse, but it largely leaves out the AIDS crisis among IV drug users, which has long been pushed to the sidelines, and urgent concerns about the transmission of HIV from parent to child. Indeed, massive resources dedicated to HIV prevention among the high-risk groups of female sex workers and men who have sex with men reproduced existing exclusions, such as invisibilization of India's border zones in the Northeast, or of trans men and lesbians.[68] Finally, this book has far more to say about the politics of prevention than about the fascinating story of the politics of treatment.[69]

OUTLINE OF THE BOOK

In order to connect the distinct scales at which this book operates, I begin and end with India's global engagements, and, in particular, with the relationship between the Indian AIDS response and the epidemic in sub-Saharan Africa. The middle chapters focus on how these global engagements shaped the lives and politics of sex workers, sexual minorities, and transgender people in Bangalore. The book moves from global fields, to the state, to organizations, and to individuals, and then it works its way back out.

Chapters 2 and 3 analyze the making of India's AIDS crisis within the global AIDS field and the Indian state's turn to civil society to meet the demands of the crisis. Chapter 2 situates the making of India's AIDS crisis within the colonial, postcolonial, and neoliberal world orders. The Indian AIDS crisis, and the scale of the state's response, was never a foregone conclusion. Rather, the Indian AIDS response, and the humanitarian resources that went with it, was generated within a global field. The chapter traces how the specter of Africa and the African epidemic, combined with postcolonial tensions about Indian sexuality, set against the immorality of the West, shaped the early Indian AIDS response. Chapter 3 analyzes the reconfiguration of Indian state agencies in response to the AIDS crisis, starting in the late 1990s. It argues that the crisis response created pockets of mutual conflict and collaboration among the state, civil society, and donors.

Chapters 4 and 5 focus on everyday experiences of the AIDS response in Bangalore, looking at how the lives and activism of sex workers and sexual minority groups changed as they engaged with the state, donors, and social movements in the heated context of a crisis. Chapter 4 focuses on NGOs, CBOs, and activist groups at the organizational level. It charts the variations that emerged among organizations linked to the AIDS response and analyzes their alliances to public health organizations and feminist, Dalit, labor, and sexual-minority activists within local political terrains. Chapter 5 shifts the focus to individual trajectories through these HIV prevention organizations. It argues that HIV prevention programs served as sites for building new forms of selfhood, through experimenting with sexual identities and discourses, gaining a stable income, and building supportive friendships.

Chapters 6 and 7 turn from the AIDS response to how it was represented. Chapter 6 begins in Bangalore and moves to Nairobi and Mombasa to examine how states and donors represented the Indian AIDS response through processes of quantification and then circulated information about it in the global AIDS field, particularly in Kenya. As the AIDS response in India was quantified, its complex political engagements were left out of the story. Chapter 7 turns to how the meanings of Indian sexuality and race were contested and reimagined as Indian AIDS programs were reformulated in Kenya. It argues that the travel of HIV prevention strategies from India to Kenya offered opportunities for relations in the global AIDS field to be reproduced, but also sometimes contested and reimagined.

Chapter 8, the conclusion, reflects on the implications of the crisis response the book analyzes, in the years after I completed the bulk of my fieldwork in 2013. Here, I return to the limits of crisis as an organizing logic for humanitarian intervention. I consider the lives of sex worker, sexual minority, and transgender activists and organizations in Bangalore as the AIDS crisis more and more became a concern of the past. The conclusion points to the conditionality of inclusion occasioned by the AIDS crisis, showing that the relationship between these stigmatized groups and state agencies was ultimately deeply precarious.

THE TEMPORALITY OF CRISIS

In the early years of India's AIDS response, writings about the topic often emphasized India's national pride and state capacity, framing AIDS as an opportunity for India to demonstrate its ability to manage a crisis effectively.[70] Today, NACO presents India's AIDS response as a success story.[71] Three decades after the first case of HIV was identified in India, then, the AIDS crisis seems like a concern of the past. Rather than uncovering the conditions of success, the aim of this book is to counter this exceptionalizing logic of crisis, to situate it within a longer trajectory of social relations, and to move from a focus on how the AIDS crisis can be solved to dissecting its political effects. As the editors of a recent volume write, AIDS is not a crisis but a "global distribution of networked *crises*"; it is an "ongoing, global crisis—experienced locally and with specificity—of enduring, structuring colonialism and racism, and all the violence to person, place, health and self-knowledge that such systems wreak."[72]

This book resituates the AIDS crisis in a longer temporal frame, as what Lauren Berlant calls *crisis ordinariness*: a view of crisis as "neither a state of exception nor the opposite, mere banality, but a domain where an upsetting scene of living is revealed to be interwoven with ordinary life after all, like ants discovered scurrying under a thoughtlessly lifted rock."[73] One interviewee, a Muslim cisgender woman sex worker I call Hajira, described a similar tension. "For our community," she said, "some . . . don't care about their health. We want to die. . . . My money has left me, my husband has left me, my children have left me, my family has left me, society itself has left me, everyone left me, why should I live?" For Hajira, the risk of HIV was only one of the everyday structures that produced her disposability, and the crisis would persist whether she protected herself from HIV or not.

One example of how crisis can be resituated is to look at how activists used the word *crisis* in their HIV prevention work. *AIDS crisis* typically refers to the threat of the disease that has killed millions of people around the world. But in the CBOs I studied in Bangalore, *crisis* had a different meaning. Sex workers, sexual minorities, and transgender people in these organizations used the word *crisis* to describe the routine challenges that emerged in their lives. *Crisis*, in this context, referred to police violence, unlawful arrest, or domestic violence, situations that were regular features of life for the sex workers, sexual minorities, and transgender people targeted by HIV prevention programs. This idea of crisis, interviewees told me, emerged when activists began to respond to calls for support from sex workers, sexual minorities, and transgender people with whom they worked. The typical understanding of *crisis* suggests the exceptionality of AIDS. Activists' use of *crisis* transformed its temporal scope. *Crisis* now referred to the enduring forms of violence that shape life at the margins of Indian political, economic, and social life. For example, activists Sunil Mohan and Rumi Harish write that "a crisis is a situation which occurs when a person is left with no support to exercise rights due to their sexual orientation and gender expression" and describe principles of crisis intervention with sex workers, sexual minorities, and transgender people that are rooted in responding to the everyday workings of patriarchy, casteism, and violence.[74] This approach to crisis, when implemented in the context of HIV prevention organizations, meant AIDS could not be isolated from the forms of exploitation and criminalization that preexisted and underpinned it.

The repurposing of *crisis* makes the fraught relationships between states, donors, and social movements particularly clear. As part of the state-funded

AIDS response, activists developed an idea of crisis that helped them to chan-
nel HIV prevention resources toward the immediate needs of sex workers,
sexual minorities, and transgender people. Later on, this idea of crisis intervention was incorporated into Gates Foundation strategy.[75] Organizations
were even required to count and report the number of crises they responded
to every month.[76] When Gates Foundation documents described crisis intervention as part of their model of HIV prevention, they did not always discuss
its origins in activist efforts and often narrowed its scope. Nevertheless, the
strategy created resources for sex workers, sexual minorities, and transgender
people to navigate criminalization and support one another.

This book's analysis of AIDS suggests a way of thinking about global
institutions rooted in an analysis of sexual politics. Global institutions are
not omnipotent; their interventions unfold within existing contexts of political mobilization and modalities of sexual governance. States mediate this
process; they are often sites of bitter struggle among activists, different state
agencies, and donors. Thinking of the state as a field, and as a battlefield,[77]
helps to make sense of these struggles. Instead of understanding the AIDS
industry as a top-down global force,[78] we can see it as a process in which states
both engage in global fields and are themselves the site of struggle. What
counts as crisis, and how the risk of crisis is managed, is ultimately political.
This meant the AIDS crisis created an opening for renegotiating gender and
sexuality. AIDS was a moment, as Patricia Hill Collins notes, to recommit
to a new sexual and gender politics.[79] Like war or natural disaster, the AIDS
crisis, even just the anticipation of it, left in its wake an altered political
terrain, with varied effects for the lives of sex workers, sexual minorities,
and transgender people.[80]

Ultimately, this book takes seriously both the material practices of the
state and social movements and the ways in which AIDS and HIV risk were
represented within global fields. AIDS is a particularly powerful example of
an immediate, urgent, life-and-death crisis whose course is fundamentally
determined by how it is defined, interpreted, represented, and governed. In
a lecture on the importance of cultural studies, Stuart Hall noted that critics
might feel unimportant during a crisis of global proportions, like AIDS. And
yet, he insisted, "the question of AIDS is an extremely important terrain of
struggle and contestation. . . . How could we say that the question of AIDS
is not also a question of who gets represented and who does not?"[81] Hall

showed that struggles over representation were life-and-death questions and that how crisis was articulated was ultimately the product of politics.[82] Hall's understanding of articulation helps illuminate how groups designated high risk, initially targets of HIV prevention, emerged from the crisis making renewed claims as citizens and linked their struggles to a range of feminist, queer, Dalit, and labor activist formations.[83]

The AIDS crisis offered a conditional form of inclusion to sex workers, sexual minorities, and transgender people. After the global AIDS crisis was assumed to be over and global institutions were no longer worried about India's AIDS epidemic, activists' relationships to global institutions grew more fragile. The link between the everyday needs of groups at risk and the imperatives of a global crisis was, then, ultimately conditional and temporary. They were included, even celebrated, for their efforts to save India from disaster, but only as long as the crisis lasted. And yet their inclusion helped distinguish India's success on a global AIDS stage, placing it in a global hierarchy of nation-states. An underlying premise of this book is that this process can tell us something about the precarious place of sexually stigmatized people in the new India. How Indian society manages sexuality is tied to the Indian state's claim to modernity. Postcolonial debates about sexuality and AIDS often lead back to questions of globalization, nationhood, and "who we are."[84] These tensions can yield contradictory opportunities for those who put the nation's sexual integrity "at risk," even when they only temporarily interrupt the conditions of their ordinariness.

2 | INDIA AND THE SPECTER OF AFRICAN AIDS

IN A 1992 EDITORIAL in the *Journal of the Indian Medical Association*, Gouri Pada Dutta, chairman of the Subject Committee on Health and Family Welfare in West Bengal, questioned the growing panic around AIDS in India. "AIDS is more a problem of the western developed countries," Dutta argued. "Africa is an exception for various reasons."[1] Dutta suggested that AIDS had not reached the numbers to qualify as a serious crisis and should not be given priority over "other diseases killing hundreds every day."[2] Speculating that this manufactured AIDS crisis might really be a "prelude to test the so-called AIDS vaccine on the Asian people," Dutta concluded that AIDS, often "described as a global problem," was in fact "being disseminated from the developed countries . . . notorious for their permissive society." In a 1995 letter, D. S. Mehra, a physician from Delhi, echoed Dutta's skepticism: "While the scientists are busy in tracing the link in the AIDS family tree we know it is a global problem that is being disseminated from the developed countries . . . the developed industrialised nations caused worldwide pollution when they bored a hole in the ozone layer. Now they are exporting HIV to the rest of the world. How these nations got the virus from African chimpanzees is a problem for the anthropologists to debate upon; we in the developing countries know where it came to us from."[3]

On the other side of skepticism and theories of Western ecological terrorism was a group of experts with a grimmer set of warnings about the Indian
AIDS crisis. In a 1994 article, Shiv Lal, the project director of the newly
formed National AIDS Control Organization, described a "really alarming"
rise in HIV prevalence in several hot spots. "The trends in Bombay, in fact,
are quite comparable to the trends earlier observed in some of the African
States like Nairobi, Adisababa [sic] from mid 80s onwards. The trends are
so similar as to forewarn us about the impending epidemic of HIV involv-
ing the general population as has happened in these African countries." In
1995, Lal coauthored an editorial in the *Indian Journal of Public Health* with
Thierry Mertens, chief of surveillance at the Global Programme on AIDS
at the WHO. Citing WHO projections, they warned that 7 million people
in India would be HIV positive by 2000 and warned against "complacency
and denial."[4] By 1996, a "frustrated" Lal had left the National AIDS Control
Programme to focus on malaria.[5]

Theories and accusations about the origins of AIDS reveal powerful insights about disease, geopolitics, and sexual imaginaries.[6] The debate centered on whether India truly was at risk of a crisis. Both sides of the debate
evoked specific symbolic and material geographies.[7] One key reference point
in this AIDS cartography was the *global*, and, more specifically, for Indian
commentators, the West. Both Dutta and Mehra argued that the global
problem of AIDS originated in Western sexual degeneracy and ecological
irresponsibility, not the developing world—indeed, they suggested that the
term *global* served to mask the Western origin of contagion. Since India was
not victim to Western sexual permissiveness, it was not at risk of an AIDS
crisis. For Lal and Mertens, by contrast, global estimates by institutions like
the WHO were key to measuring the future of India's AIDS epidemic against
the barriers of Indian complacency. Global quantitative measures indexed
technical prowess and political neutrality and lent urgency to the WHO's
predictions of an Indian AIDS crisis.

A second reference point that emerged in these debates was Africa.[8]
For critics preoccupied with the evils of the West, the African origins of
AIDS were a distracting preoccupation that masked a plot to test vaccines
in the developing world. For other experts, in contrast, Africa—a reference that collapsed all variation in African countries' AIDS epidemics into

one—represented the worst of what the Indian epidemic could become. It provided a dire forewarning of India's future.[9] While scholars have written about the postcolonial binaries of Western and Indian sexuality that shaped representations of AIDS in India at different points in the epidemic, less has been written about the idea of Africa that simultaneously shaped the early Indian response to AIDS.[10] But, as the sociologist Cindy Patton writes, global imaginaries of AIDS can be "mapped directly on to pre-existing national and cultural formations," within which the idea of Africa as the source and epitome of the AIDS crisis plays a central role.[11] AIDS entails claims to both "the international community" and to the nation.[12] By broadening the symbolic map on which discourses of Indian sexuality play out, this chapter offers a way of thinking through not only postcolonial national discourses of tradition and purity that commentators used to distinguish India from the West but also racialized discourses of modernity, morality, and civilizational advancement that shaped how experts distinguished India from Africa.[13]

The shifting relationships between India, Africa, and the West form the symbolic backdrop against which experts calculated infection risk, assessed sexual cultures, and designed response strategies in the first decade of the Indian AIDS response. This chapter argues that these relations among nation-states were central to how the AIDS crisis was defined and managed in India. Within the global AIDS field, India was positioned materially and symbolically in contrast to other states and especially against the US and Africa. India's status as at risk of a devastating crisis was defined within this set of relationships: Africa represented the crisis, and India was at risk of one. This status had monetary consequences: the World Bank provided US$84 million for the first National AIDS Control Programme starting in 1992 on the assumption that India was at risk of a large-scale epidemic. AIDS institutions formed a global platform on which the modern Indian state distinguished itself from both Western sexual permissiveness and the devastating future of those African states that were already facing an AIDS catastrophe. These relationships also had consequences for how experts conceptualized the epidemic and crafted policy. Through a postcolonial circuit of scientific evidence from Africa to India, mediated by UN and other global institutions, the prostitute[14] came to be understood as the heart of the crisis.

Scholars of international development point to a shared social space that NGOs, donors, global governance institutions including UN agencies and the World Bank, bilateral aid agencies including USAID and the British Department for International Development (DfID), and national governments occupy.[15] Within this shared social space—one this book refers to as a field—actors need not share an orientation, but they are "oriented toward each other in formulating their differences."[16] In the field, each works to create the next success story to achieve global recognition, the next best practice or model for other countries,[17] or the next big grant from a major corporate philanthropist. Risk was defined within a global field: experts warned that India was facing what commentators called an "Africa-like"[18] AIDS trajectory.

Scholarship in public health and medicine is a revealing index of the debates and conflicts surrounding India's position in the global AIDS field and the changing understandings of its relative risk. This chapter analyzes articles in the public health and medical literature, in both Indian and US medical journals, to draw out the debates that shaped the early years of India's AIDS crisis. References to the foreign, both Western and African, suffuse the early medical scholarship about the arrival of AIDS in India. To situate these debates within popular discourse at the time, my analysis also draws on a selection of articles in the English-language press from the *Times of India* and the *New York Times*. I also draw on interdisciplinary feminist scholarship on colonial sexual regulation and disease control in India.

Global fields have colonial histories,[19] and development and humanitarian fields offer a clear example. International NGOs like Oxfam formed just as the British Empire was beginning to disintegrate, and the concept of development was first put into practice by colonial officials hoping to retain their hold on political authority.[20] Understanding the contemporary stakes of public health crisis in India, then, requires an understanding of the colonial history of sexual crisis. This chapter follows three historical moments to demonstrate how discourses of India's sexual crises have been produced within a global field. First, in the late nineteenth century, the Contagious Diseases Acts laid the groundwork for Indian health officials' approach to sexually transmitted disease and crystallized the link between native sexuality, disease, and national moral character. Second, in the mid-1980s, postcolonial nationalist understandings of Western homosexuality and Indian and African heterosexuality shaped debates about whether AIDS posed a threat to India or not. Third, by the mid-1990s, when the WHO began warning of India's impending AIDS crisis, drawing on epidemiological models based on research done in Africa, warnings that India must avoid an Africa-like epidemic became increasingly strident. Through all three moments, the prostitute or sex worker emerged as central to disease control. Ultimately, whether India was at risk of an AIDS crisis or not was never a simple quantitative truth. It was tied up with struggles over the character of Indian sexuality. And these questions, in turn, were fundamentally shaped by discourses of sovereignty and Western domination, tradition and modernity, and Indianness and Africanness—questions of where India fit into the colonial, postcolonial, and neoliberal world orders.

SEX, DISEASE, AND REGULATION IN LATE COLONIALISM

Long before AIDS, in the late nineteenth century, the regulation of sexual crisis crystallized tensions around race, sexuality, and empire. The colonial Contagious Diseases Act was passed in British Parliament in 1864 and extended in 1866 and 1869. Together, the acts responded to a rise in venereal disease in the British military by regulating prostitution.[21] The 1864 Cantonment Acts and the 1868 Indian Contagious Diseases Act expanded this regulation of prostitution to India. As the historian Philippa Levine shows, the Contagious Diseases Acts ultimately reflected "the need to bring to heel sexual disorder among colonized peoples;" "health thus became a moral and a national problem."[22] The association of sexual deviance with lack of moral hygiene, with venereal disease as the result, lay at the heart of colonial ideas about racial hierarchy.[23] The disordered sexuality of colonized people formed a contrast to British morality and civilizational superiority and was the target of repeated efforts at reform.

The Contagious Diseases Acts centered on the prostitute rather than the soldier. The prostitute was a vexed figure for British colonial officials. Scholarship on various parts of ancient and medieval South Asia describes a rich and varied tradition in which exchanges of sex and money were integrated into political and religious life.[24] For late nineteenth-century British administrators, these varied traditions formed a site of fascination and discomfort, and they were often the target of regulation. Both sexologists and colonial administrators solidified the prostitute as a stable concept that became central to their understanding of civilizational hierarchy and social deviance.[25] At the same time, the British military presence was closely intertwined with prostitution and the brothel industry in major Indian cities.[26] Instead of seeking to eradicate prostitution, the acts mandated its regulation, with a system of mandatory disease checks and *lock hospitals* to detain and treat women found to have venereal disease.

The acts were controversial from the start, and the vocal resistance they elicited from white British women highlighted tensions about race and sexual character. Josephine Butler, who cofounded the Ladies' National Association for the Repeal of the Contagious Diseases Acts in Britain and later turned her attention to India, saw the acts as condoning and enabling immorality in the British troops and thus as a stain on the moral leadership of the British Empire. The Indian Contagious Diseases Act was not repealed until 1888, two years after the acts were repealed in Great Britain, and lock hospitals continued to be used for longer, through the 1890s.[27] After 1886, British women reformers turned their attention to India.[28] They protested colonial officials' role in tolerating and regulating immorality. White women reformers also wrote of native women's suffering at the hands of corrupt British soldiers. Two visiting American reformers, Elizabeth Andrew and Katherine Bushnell, for example, called for readers to "weigh the soul of . . . one dark-skinned heathen against the diseased bodies of a standing army of men" and asked, "shall it be immorality and medicine, or shall it be morality?"[29] At the heart of these accounts, whether they depicted Indian prostitutes as diseased and degenerate or innocent sufferers of British male vice, lies the concern that regulated Indian prostitution threatened morality and, in particular, the ethical authority of the white Empire.

While the Contagious Diseases Acts largely focused their regulatory attention on the diseased and/or suffering female prostitute and argued for regulation or abolition, the threat of homosexuality ran through the debates over them. Preventing homosexuality in the British troops was a key objective of regulating prostitution. Male prostitution alarmed British officials, as did sex between male British soldiers. Regulated prostitution with women became the lesser evil.[30] More generally, colonial officials saw both homosexuality and prostitution as symptoms of native immorality, which they regulated through a range of mechanisms. In both Britain and the colonies, homosexuality was criminalized as unnatural: the 1860 Indian Penal Code criminalized sodomy (or "carnal intercourse against the order of nature"), and the 1885 Criminal Law Amendment Act in Britain both criminalized "gross indecency" between men and increased criminal penalties against brothel-keepers.[31] Medical practices played a key role in the documentation and adjudication of sexual crimes.[32] Ultimately, ideas of deviant sexuality animated images of natives as "queer and uncivilized."[33] As with colonial anxieties over prostitution, anxieties over homosexuality ultimately hinged on controlling unruly native sexuality, a source of curiosity and fear for colonial officials, especially when it threatened to become, biologically or figuratively, contagious.

Late nineteenth-century battles over contagious disease provide important context for the debates over the AIDS crisis a century later. The battle lines that emerged—between tolerating (but pathologizing) deviant Indian sexuality and seeking to eradicate it on moral grounds—would re-emerge in battles in the mid-2000s over decriminalizing homosexuality and sex work. When Gloria Steinem visited Calcutta, where sex worker collectives ran HIV prevention programs, and "was ashamed to see 'sex worker,' the only English words amid Bengali, on signs in Sonagachi," her indignation recalled the outrage of American and British women reformers in the late nineteenth century who decried colonial medical authorities in India for regulating instead of abolishing prostitution.[34] Colonial debates over the Contagious Diseases Acts linked sexuality and the management of disease to the moral character of the race. When AIDS arrived in India, the ensuing debates revived this colonial symbolic architecture.

INDIAN HETEROSEXUALITY, FOREIGN INFLUENCES, AND THE ARRIVAL OF AIDS IN THE MID-1980S

If British colonial officials largely positioned venereal diseases as native sexual contagion, postcolonial Indian commentators in the 1980s saw them as a mark of Western vice. In 1985, though AIDS cases had not yet been documented in India, reports of AIDS elsewhere, especially in the US, began to attract attention in the Indian media. Visits from US experts put AIDS on the radar for the Indian medical establishment. But they mostly described AIDS as a foreign threat. Pearl Ma, a microbiologist at St. Vincent's in New York, told reporters in Bombay that "the disease could have already found its way into the country through tourists."[35] Halfdan Mahler, director general of the WHO, announced in Bangalore that "seventy percent of AIDS victims were located in the US and the rest in western countries."[36] Other visiting experts, mostly from the US, warned against importing blood for blood transfusions and risking HIV transmission.[37]

This association of AIDS with the West was often linked, in Indian media reports, to dismissing homosexuality as a Western indulgence. J. K. Maniar, president of the Indian Association for the Study of Sexually Transmitted Diseases, told the press that the "homosexuality percentage" in India was "five to 15 per cent homosexuals," compared to "40 to 60 per cent" in the US. He added that "the possibility of AIDS spreading to India are further reduced thanks to our society, which has imposed sexual taboos, making sexual promiscuity like pre-marital sex or heterosexuality [sic] quite uncommon." Nevertheless, he warned that "with the influence of western culture . . . the youth are being drawn into a style of free-living which, if unchecked, could prove quite harmful."[38] These ideas of AIDS, and homosexuality, as foreign were soon reflected in preventative measures. In West Bengal, the health minister and the mayor of Calcutta ordered an investigation of AIDS, including "the purchase of used garments from abroad" (which had already been banned in Bangladesh in Pakistan) and the dangers of "sailors from abroad."[39] An article in the *Journal of the Indian Medical Association* argued that prevention efforts must begin in earnest—first, because India was ill-equipped to deal with the an epidemic the way the US and other wealthy countries could and, second, because of the looming threat of foreign sexual practices within India. "Apart from normal sexual practice, the so-called perverted sexual procedures, viz, homosexuality, drug abuse and habit of taking the intravenous narcotic drugs are not unknown in the present Indian society. Quite a good section of people, especially the rich and the higher middle classes of the major cities, are fond of imitating the life-style of the western world."[40] These accounts mapped the movement of AIDS from West to East but suggested that, for the most part, "Indians are normally saved from such diseases" because of their "conservative value system and single partner sex life," as opposed to the "indiscriminate homosexuality [of] the westerners."[41] Activists pointed to the contradictions of these evocations of Indian purity. "No sex, please, we're Indian," jokes a cartoon about this initial response in Siddharth Dube's book *Sex, Lies and AIDS*.[42]

These accounts of AIDS as a Western affliction crystallized the aspirations and tensions of postcolonial nationhood. Reports in both the Indian and US media sought to characterize the main mechanisms of the Indian epidemic and position them in a global context. Ideas of India as a poor and rural nation, sexually moral except for the threat of a Westernized and potentially homosexual elite,[43] reflected, in part, Cold War geopolitics.[44] (The *Times of India* also reported, for example, that Russia was "untouched by AIDS," quoting Russian officials who dismissed AIDS as a product of Western licentiousness.)[45] This idea of AIDS as Western began to shift as AIDS cases began to be identified on the subcontinent. Once a case of AIDS was reported in Pakistan, the Indian Council of Medical Research set up a task force and began importing diagnostic kits for HIV testing.[46] India's first AIDS clinic opened in Bombay in March 1986.[47]

Commentary on India's imperviousness to AIDS shifted decisively in the mid-1980s. In April of 1986, the Union health minister announced in Parliament that six women in Tamil Nadu had been confirmed to have AIDS.[48] "AIDS has set foot on Indian soil, the devastating firmness of which would be felt in coming years," wrote one *Times of India* reader from Bombay.[49] Another warned that AIDS "may ultimately lead to extinction of mankind" and noted that the six women "the fact that this baffling disease has originated mainly in countries like the US, USSR, Britain, France, West Germany and Italy, shows that it is a curse from God for their sinful deeds of squandering huge sums of money on weapons of destruction in the very face of billions of people dying due to hunger in large parts of the world."[50] The *Times of India* reported that the six women "were known to be of promiscuous behavior" but that they "had no history of contact with white people, though they had contacts with foreigners."[51] In these accounts, the women's deviant sexuality became a site for the entry of foreign contagion.

The allusion to foreigners who were not white hints at a shift in the geography of AIDS discourses in the mid-1980s. Fears of the Western origin of AIDS were gradually replaced with a vision of the AIDS epidemic coming from a different source—Africa. In 1985, at both the first International AIDS Conference in Atlanta and an infectious disease conference in Cairo, experts warned of an African epidemic that was largely heterosexual, and the announcement caught the attention of the Indian media.[52] The *Times of India* reported that AIDS was "widely prevalent in Zaire, Ruanda [*sic*], Burundi, Kenya, Uganda and Tanzania" but had not yet arrived in Asia.[53] It reported an African origin to the disease, beginning with African green monkeys and then spreading by "the practice of using a single needle for giving injections to many patients" and "free sex among the rural population."[54] It was easier to dismiss stories of Western sexual permissiveness fanning the flames of an

AIDS explosion than to dismiss the threat of "a lethal epidemic throughout the crowded cities and villages of the third world."[55]

As the epidemic progressed, the idea of India's potential similarity to Africa became increasingly ubiquitous, and the role of female prostitutes was a central point of comparison. Research published in *The Lancet* in January 1987 confirmed expectations that India's was a heterosexual epidemic, largely spread through heterosexual contact, and that female prostitutes and female STD clinic attendees were the main risk groups.[56] This confirmation of AIDS cases in India attracted international attention. The first article in the *New York Times* about AIDS in India, published in February 1987, reported seventy-one cases of AIDS, with a "high number of women who are prostitutes among the total" (about fifty-one of the seventy-one cases). It noted, but only in passing, that five Indian men who had likely contracted AIDS in Europe and North America had died in the last year. It ended by noting that "AIDS is believed to be spread predominantly by heterosexual transmission in Africa."[57] Associating India's epidemic with Africa's epidemic, largely heterosexual and contained among female prostitutes, except for a small Westernized homosexual elite, helped medical authorities confirm their assumption that homosexuality was foreign to Indian sexuality. India's epidemic was a heterosexual epidemic, like the epidemic in Africa, and not a homosexual one, like the one in the West.[58]

Documenting further AIDS cases in prostitutes helped further dismiss the possibility of a homosexual epidemic. The early surveillance efforts functioned as a self-fulfilling prophecy. In the 1987 article in *The Lancet*, for example, the authors report that they tested 1,025 female prostitutes for HIV, of whom thirty—or 2.9%—were positive, and seventy homosexual men for HIV, of whom none were positive. Though they conclude that "the mode of spread is predominantly via heterosexual contact," the much smaller number of homosexual men they studied largely predisposed the conclusion.[59] A few deaths from AIDS in elite and Westernized gay men, it seemed, could be overlooked, but the real crisis would arrive when AIDS hit the general population. This process would be mediated, as in Africa, by female prostitutes.

If the real risk of an Indian AIDS epidemic lay in heterosexual prostitution, and if the Indian epidemic were more similar to African epidemics than Western ones, two groups would draw the bulk of regulatory attention: sex workers and Africans,[60] or, as it appeared more euphemistically in *Nature*, a "pool of infected women"[61] and "foreign students."[62] The two groups soon faced repressive measures. Recalling the administrative mechanisms used under the Contagious Diseases Acts, medical authorities detained sex workers for mandatory testing and confinement. And Africans in India faced heightened restrictions on entering the country. In 1986, *Nature* reported that India had thirty thousand foreign students, "mostly from Africa and eastern Asia."[63] After an African student was found to be HIV positive,[64] the Indian Ministry of Health announced in October 1986 that AIDS testing was compulsory for all foreign students seeking admission to Indian universities.[65] African students protested the racist guidelines by boycotting the test,[66] and in February 1987, African students organized a protest march in Delhi, arguing that the testing constituted medical apartheid.[67] Nevertheless, by March 1987, eleven African students thought to be HIV-positive had been deported.[68]

These repressive measures made particularly clear that Africans, and not Western foreigners, now faced the brunt of regulatory attention on preventing the foreign threat of AIDS. In general, the Indian state did not restrict temporary travelers from the West in the name of AIDS.[69] Attempts to restrict the behavior of Western foreigners were usually met with wide disapproval. In 1988, A. S. Paintal, the director-general of the Indian Council of Medical Research (ICMR), asked the Ministry of Health to ban sex with all foreigners. The proposed penalty, imposed on the Indian citizen not the foreigner, would be ₹20,000 and three months in jail. The statement was controversial; the Ministry of Law opposed it. The *Indian Express* said it would "offend human dignity," and *India Today* called it "absurd."[70] On the other hand, foreign students, a category which usually implied Africans, could be deported for being HIV positive. Even in the face of international media attention, Prime Minister Narasimha Rao refused to change the guidelines facing African students. The rules remained in place through the 1990s and were lifted only in 2002.[71] In 1990, an African diplomat was refused surgery at the All India Institute of Medical Sciences after he tested HIV positive and died a few days later.[72]

The early response to the arrival of AIDS in India set the stage for later battles over India's AIDS crisis. Was AIDS a problem for India, or was it mainly a problem of the West? If India did face an AIDS crisis, would it unfold like the AIDS crisis in Africa? And what did these relationships say about

Indian sexuality? In short, the AIDS crisis demanded that Indian medical authorities position Indian sexuality within a global AIDS field. The medical consensus settled on the conclusion that India's sexual norm was heterosexual and monogamous, not "permissive" and homosexual like the West. Experts now sought to distinguish India not from the West but from Africa. To stop an African-style epidemic before it started, they both contained sex workers and prevented Africans from entering the country.

Importantly, these developments unfolded in the context of a rise in right-wing Hindu nationalist discourses that positioned gender and sexuality as key sites for battles over Hindu morality in contrast to dangerous Western values. Both Africans and sex workers—stereotyped as hypersexual and dangerous to this nationalist morality—were marked as a risk.[73] The external risk to the nation—of an Africa-like epidemic—was now imagined onto the bodies of the risky groups *within* the nation. This battle over India's place in the global AIDS field, the importance of distinguishing India from Africa, and the urgency of regulating internal others would gain heightened relevance in the 1990s, when WHO experts began to warn that India was the next epicenter of the AIDS epidemic.

AFRICA'S PRESENT, INDIA'S FUTURE, AND
THE AIDS PANIC OF THE 1990S

By the early 1990s, warnings of a neglected crisis in India mounted, in particular from the WHO. European and North American AIDS experts argued that the Indian government was ignoring what they suggested was destined to become the next epicenter of the AIDS epidemic. While officials within NACO were corroborating these WHO warnings, critics were contesting them, arguing that the Indian AIDS crisis was manufactured by the West and was monopolizing funds and political attention.

As experts drew increasing attention to the Indian AIDS epidemic, the specter of Africa played an increasingly prominent role. Statistical projections about the future of the epidemic depended on information from existing epidemics, so numbers from Africa were often the starting point.[74] These projections positioned Asia as the next frontier of the African AIDS epidemic and defined India's risk in relation to Africa.[75] The AIDS activist Siddharth Dube warned that "Africa's present HIV/AIDS-caused hell is very probably India's future."[76]

Building on comparisons to African epidemics, the WHO's projections for the Indian AIDS epidemic grew increasingly dire. In 1990, the WHO told the ICMR that HIV was being transmitted heterosexually in India and that India would face at least sixty-thousand AIDS cases by 1995. Paintal said these WHO projections should not be dismissed, and that India was entering a "disaster phase."[77] These warnings circulated in the global medical literature. *The Lancet* reported in 1990 that "the picture is looking very gloomy. . . . The early suggestions that the spread of the disease would be contained because Indian society is sexually conservative have proved to be self deluding."[78] A 1991 *British Medical Journal* article reported that "While the AIDS epidemic may be slowing in Western countries, the view to the east [India and Thailand] is threatening." The article quoted Vulimiri Ramalingaswami, from the All India Institute of Medical Sciences, as noting that "In India we are sitting on top of a volcano."[79] Even the *New York Times* reported that "In an Unaware India, AIDS Threat Is Growing."[80] In 1992, Michael Merson, director of the Global AIDS Programme at the WHO, told *The Lancet* that "the prevalence of HIV infection in India could reach that in Africa if spread of the infection is not limited within the next three years."[81] A *Times of India* article captured the temporal geography that linked India to the US and Africa: "The AIDS epidemic, cutting its deathly swathe across the world, has moved from the gay communities of San Francisco and entire populations in sub-Saharan Africa to fill in its ominous shadow lines throughout the Asia-Pacific region."[82]

On the other hand, skepticism remained, with Indian medical journals an instructive example. In the *Journal of the Indian Medical Association,* a Calcutta psychiatrist wrote that "Many hazards are perceived to be more threatening and fatal than they really are. . . . we are building castles of acquired immunodeficiency syndrome (AIDS) prevention in the air. . . . This is the paradox of medical preaching of colonial culture to which we are still subjugated."[83] Arabinda Chowdhury argued that India's limited socioeconomic conditions and "other prevailing and preventable fatal diseases" as well as "the basic needs of human life" meant that AIDS prevention was "an expensive luxury."[84] Detailing the struggles of overburdened public health systems in Tanzania, Zaire, and Rwanda to keep up with AIDS costs, Chowdhury argued for an approach to HIV that focused on prevention within broader socioeconomic conditions. L. R. Murmu, from the All India Institute of Medical Sciences, echoed this argument in a letter to *The Lancet,* saying that AIDS strategies would be "meaningless" without addressing "social problems" and "political conditions."[85] These commentators were skeptical of rich countries imposing unreasonable pressure to address AIDS on a poor country that lacked the wealth for a large-scale disease response. Some even questioned WHO projections. For example, a letter to the *Times of India* speculated that the WHO had not reported on any Indian AIDS cases and argued that "AIDS mania" was ill founded.[86]

Wariness of global institutions grew particularly pronounced with the announcement of the Indian government's first National AIDS Control Programme for 1992–1997, a US$100 million program, of which $84.5 million would come from the World Bank. The funds constituted 15% of India's health budget, behind only malaria in allocation, and more than three times the funds allotted for tuberculosis. I. S. Gilada of the Indian Health Organisation criticized the program for reserving 19% of funds for foreign consultants and 40% for an intermediary agency.[87] L. R. Murmu argued that this conditional assistance "does not reflect the spirit of so-called extraordinary co-operation" and criticized the "reliance of these programmes on the wisdom of donor countries."[88] The Indian government remained cautious in permitting vaccine trials by US researchers in Indian clinics. "Most of the sites are in African countries with histories of similar work and little chance of opposition," wrote reporters for *Nature*. "India, however, has until recently been skeptical of collaborations with US scientists."[89] To these reporters, Africa offered a different kind of warning—not of an unchecked epidemic but of excessive deference to US scientists.

These debates began to come to a head in 1994 and 1995, when the first National AIDS Control Programme (NACP I) came under increased national and global scrutiny. In 1994, India's health minister admitted to Parliament that NACP I had run up against a number of challenges, and that the $100 million budget had been underutilized.[90] A WHO report argued that World Bank funds were being "misused." Condoms were being used to plug up leaking radiators on trucks[91] or being melted down for use by toy manufacturers.[92] An article in a global AIDS journal noted that "India has no room for complacency."[93] Sriram Prasad Tripathy, A WHO consultant, formerly of the ICMR, described the AIDS program as "a bloody mess."[94]

In the face of these critiques of the Indian government's lackluster AIDS response, estimates of India's looming epidemic grew even larger. In a 1994 article, "Dallying with Death: The Impending Crisis in India," which won an award at the International AIDS Conference in Yokohama, Jaya Shreedhar wrote, "To the average Indian strolling down the street or shopping in a crowded marketplace, things appear perfectly normal, whereas chances are that one or more people around him are infected with HIV."[95] These accounts of latent crisis encouraged fears of pathological sexual immorality lurking just beneath the surface of everyday life, a crisis that was imminent even if it didn't look like it. Gilada predicted that 2 million people in India were already HIV positive and 30 million to 50 million people in India would be HIV positive by 2000.[96] World Bank documents predicted 37 million HIV-positive Indians by 2005.[97]

Epidemiological estimates supported these warnings of impending crisis and continued to grow in urgency, often referencing patterns of transmission in Africa. For example, a 1995 article in the *American Journal of Epidemiology* proposed a new method of estimating HIV incidence and concluded that HIV incidence in Pune could have been underestimated by as much as 60%. It argued that India's epidemic had a doubling time "similar to doubling times reported in the 1980s in selected populations in a number of countries in Africa, such as Malawi, Kenya, and Uganda."[98] A 1995 review study led by Robert Bollinger, an epidemiologist at Johns Hopkins Medical School, predicted that India would have 5 million HIV-positive people by 2000, the largest number of HIV-positive people in the world. Bollinger and colleagues noted that HIV seroprevalence rates in Indian sex workers "are rivaling those reported among homosexual men of the early 1980s in the United States and among [commercial sex workers] and STD clinic patients in Africa during the mid-1980s." To these US experts, these numbers suggested "the inevitable spread of HIV to other segments of the general population, as documented in Africa and other areas of the world," with "catastrophic" consequences.[99]

In global medical journals, the language of crisis grew widespread. Headlines like "AIDS in Position to Ravage India,"[100] "HIV and India: Looking into the Abyss,"[101] and "India AIDS Situation Seen Out of Control by 2000"[102] captured a sense of looming catastrophe. On the first day of the International AIDS Conference in Vancouver in 1996, Peter Piot, the head of the newly formed UN AIDS program, UNAIDS, announced that India had 3 million people living with HIV. The *New York Times* headline indicated the shock of the announcement: "India Suddenly Leads in H.I.V., AIDS Meeting Is

Told."[103] The UNAIDS/WHO *Report on the Global HIV/AIDS Epidemic June 1998* reported that now 4 million people in India were living with HIV.[104] A report in the *New York Times* described India as "the world center of the disease by the end of the century," when 10 million to even 50 million people would have HIV. The article noted that nationalists and other critics remained "blinded" by denial and a refusal to take estimates seriously.[105] These reports even provoked US security concerns. India's large population, US commentators noted, meant that a large-scale AIDS epidemic there could "derail the economic prospects of billions" and "alter the global military balance."[106]

Debates in Indian media and medical journals in this period revealed that the determination of risk was deeply contested. While some excoriated the government's "suicidal complacency" and warned that "we in India are sitting on a biological time bomb,"[107] others warned against the "unnecessary panic," "scare propaganda," and "wild statements" produced by the WHO, the ICMR, and morally suspect "globalized media."[108] Journalist Sadhna Mohan wrote that "the AIDS scare in India could be aid-induced" and challenged the US media for quoting the WHO's unfounded estimates and NACO for failing to provide an alternative. The scholar Ritu Priya argued that the "panic reaction" would perpetuate stigma.[109] But both sides of the debate over whether India faced an AIDS crisis or not placed India within a field in relation to the West and Africa. While critics suggested that India was distinct from Africa and thus not at risk of crisis, those who feared the AIDS epidemic placed India within a temporal and spatial map of the epidemic in which Africa represented the worst of what India could become.

FROM KENYA TO INDIA

As the 1990s wore on, the projections of an explosive epidemic increasingly won out over the skepticism. The budget for the National AIDS Control Programme quadrupled in its second phase, starting in 1999, and reached US$2.5 billion in its third phase, starting in 2003.[110] This shift unfolded through debates among Indian medical experts, state agencies, donors, and global institutions over whether India's epidemic was following the path of AIDS in Africa. These epidemiological debates were translated into projects and programs through institutional relationships that applied epidemiological assumptions from Africa to the Indian context.[111] Researchers traveled between Africa and India, using techniques of measurement, intervention, and evaluation from Africa to aid in managing India's encounter with AIDS. Epidemiological expertise developed in the Kenyan epidemic was a key conduit in this transnational circuit.

When I interviewed the director of an HIV prevention program for men in sex work in Nairobi, in 2013, he told me he was surprised to learn that "India actually learned from Kenya." Researchers, he explained, had once drawn on Kenyan approaches in responding to the Indian epidemic. Canadian researchers' presence in Nairobi dated back to the early 1980s, when they began studying HIV resistance among a group of sex workers. One epidemiologist who would go on to design large-scale studies and eventually coordinate programs across Karnataka explained in an interview that "the Kenya approach was definitely a basis for us." Studies done in Kenya became the basis for larger-scale interventions in India: "Kenya was a research project. Now [in India] it's programming." Researchers who had developed their understanding of HIV in Nairobi became part of the planning process for HIV prevention efforts in India, especially in Karnataka.

Through these research connections, the centrality of female prostitutes to the Indian AIDS epidemic solidified. One of the key mechanisms researchers identified in their research in Kenya and applied to the Indian epidemic was the categorization of high-risk groups. Among the first studies of AIDS in sub-Saharan Africa were studies of female prostitutes in Nairobi.[112] A group of Canadian researchers in Nairobi had begun studying STDs in the neighborhood of a large STD clinic in the late 1970s, and they were the first to announce the arrival of HIV in East Africa in 1986 in a widely cited article in the *New England Journal of Medicine*.[113] These studies were used to establish the prevalence of disease and prove that the epidemic in sub-Saharan Africa, unlike in North America, was fueled by heterosexual transmission.[114]

The prostitute was by no means a simple category to define in Nairobi. Nairobi's early urban development was driven by migrant workers supported by various types of reproductive labor, including prostitution.[115] The influential Kenyan studies focused on visible urban prostitution, but not the wide range of sexual exchanges that took place in the city. Researchers themselves explained that they studied Nairobi prostitutes, in part, because they were "readily identifiable."[116] As Karen Booth shows, these researchers developed a model of AIDS spread through female sex workers and mobile migrant male truck drivers. In this model, prostitutes formed the *reservoir* of disease.[117] In these studies, the category of the prostitute, as Booth points out, was poorly defined; who counted as a prostitute was unclear and more often defined by neighborhood than by practice. Sometimes, a man simply reporting that he had contracted HIV from a prostitute was taken to be evidence of the epidemic spreading through prostitution. These categories nevertheless became central to how AIDS was understood and tracked in both sub-Saharan Africa and India. When researchers moved to India, they applied the same models of prostitutes and truck drivers as vectors of the epidemic that they had developed in Kenya. These models built on an existing pattern of social scientific governance that, as Durba Mitra argues, reified the prostitute—and deviant feminine sexuality—as the locus of social ills.[118]

It is not particularly unusual that epidemiologists drew from the information they had available to make sense of an impending epidemic. But these institutional relationships show how determinations of risk are formed in a global field in which statistical models and discourses travel and local conditions are mapped. Ideas about India's similarities and differences from Africa and the West shaped which kinds of evidence and models of transmission were produced and considered relevant. Prevention strategies, and the political formations they inadvertently became part of, ensued from these foundational assumptions.

THE MAKING AND UNMAKING OF CRISIS

After over a decade of statements from the WHO and UNAIDS about India's denialism and refusal to engage with its ticking time bomb of an AIDS epidemic, the panic about AIDS in India began to subside in the mid-2000s. In 2005, UNAIDS estimated that 5.7 million people were living with HIV in India, a number that still indicated the largest HIV burden in the world.[119] NACO countered, arguing that its estimates suggested only 5.2 million people living with HIV in the country.[120] Two years later, NACO and UNAIDS announced unexpected news: the estimate had been revised to 2.4 million.[121] Drawing on new survey data and estimation methodologies, researchers found that the AIDS crisis in India was far less explosive than previously thought.

The revision provoked renewed debate. The findings vindicated critics of the apocalyptic estimates of the 1990s and the Indian health officials who saw global institutions as creating unnecessary panic in India. And they worried both activists and donors, like the Gates Foundation, who had relied on big numbers to draw attention and funding to their work.[122] The revised estimates suggested that India's epidemic was not like those in southern Africa after all. India's HIV prevalence had remained relatively low outside at-risk groups; the predicted spread to the general population had never arrived.

Nevertheless, the dramatic estimates in the 1980s and 1990s put India on the epidemiological map for its part in the global AIDS crisis. India's relationship to the West and Africa informed the policy decisions of Indian AIDS officials as the epidemic progressed. The Indian AIDS response remained predominantly focused, in its early years, on female sex workers, and public health campaigns urged men to remain within the bounds of monogamous marriage. But men who have sex with men—not to mention trans women—were rendered largely invisible in epidemiological estimates of India's "heterosexual epidemic" and were far less acknowledged by the national AIDS response until the mid-2000s.[123] This neglect persisted despite continuous activist efforts to face up to the criminalization and stigmatization of homosexuality as core drivers of HIV transmission.[124] In the US, critical scholars of AIDS have noted that the gentrification of memories of AIDS activism erases the experiences of sex workers and Black and Latinx people[125] in the shadows of a presumed white, elite, cis-male, gay epidemic.[126] In an obverse way, epidemiological characterizations of India's heterosexual epidemic driven by female sex workers helped reinforce the idea that there was no such thing as Indian homosexuality. By analyzing media and public health accounts of Western, Indian, and African epidemics, this chapter has shown how these erasures emerged in relation to one another.

The making of India's AIDS crisis highlights the intricate ways in which India participated in this global field. Nationalist skeptics suggested that the AIDS crisis had been manufactured by global institutions, imposing their will on India in a scheme to win profits on vaccine development or expensive fees for foreign public health consultants. Some accounts of the AIDS industry might suggest a similarly coercive process of medical surveillance driven by US donors. But this chapter has traced a more complex (and more multiscalar) process. The AIDS crisis was not manufactured solely by global institutions. Instead, it emerged through relationships between global institutions and Indian ones. Actors within the national public health field exploited alignments with the global AIDS field to advance their cause.[127] Indian NGO leaders like Gilada of the Indian Health Organisation, Anjali Gopalan of the Naz Foundation, and Smarajit Jana of the Durbar Mahila Samanwaya Committee were quoted in the international media arguing for the urgency of the crisis, and state officials like Shiv Lal, the director of NACO, insisted that AIDS should not be dismissed. These NGO leaders leveraged their global links to push for attention to AIDS within India and to open space for negotiation with the state around questions of sexuality.

Once India's AIDS epidemic had been globally recognized as a crisis, the Indian state faced the daunting task of managing it. But its limited bu-reaucratic reach, combined with the criminalization of the targeted groups of sex workers, sexual minorities, and transgender people it most needed to involve, meant that the state needed to suspend typical procedure and create alternative spaces and strategies for HIV prevention. Faced with these contradictions, the state turned to activists and NGOs, as well as global donors and institutions, to help manage the crisis. This strategy began with a logic of containing and isolating risk but gradually became the grounds for incorporating high-risk groups into narrowly defined state programs. The next chapter examines the conflicts and collaborations produced by this conjuncture.

3 | FROM CONTAINMENT
TO INCORPORATION

I ARRIVED A BIT AFTER NOON to a training event for brothel madams on the terrace of an old house. Chandra, from the CBO organizing the training, had told me everything would be over by eleven, but I knew by then not to worry too much about being late. A few of us sipped mango juice and chatted while we waited for others to arrive. The attendees arrived together and settled into rows of chairs in front of a small podium, decorated with a brightly colored awning. After a quick icebreaker—a role-play about a tiger in the forest who learns he needs the other animals to help him—a young man from another organization began a lecture about the causes and prevention of HIV. "Who knows how to use a condom?" he asked, with didactic flair. Everyone raised their hand. "We're all people who know it, sir," someone called out. "Let's talk about how to do it anyway," he said. "Sometimes people don't really know how to do it, even if they say they do." One at a time, he called on four volunteers from the audience. Each executed a flawless demonstration of how to put a condom on a standard-issue, bright-red model of a penis. Nevertheless, the man gave an additional demonstration himself, sitting on a chair with the model carefully positioned between his knees. I heard some suppressed laughter and raised my hand. "Say we know how to use a condom perfectly. I ask a client to use a condom and he says no. What do I do?" The demonstrator looked up from the condom. "You have to make him understand.

Explain to him that's for the good of both of you." "He might still say no!" one of the madams said, laughing. "Explain it to him," he repeated. Chandra nudged me and whispered in my ear. "For that question, come to our office. I'll show you. We do role-plays." The demonstrator moved on.

Over lunch, the peer educators complained about the training. "I've heard it a million times, the same story," one said. "But this is what the project is!" said someone else. "You can't go outside of that." After lunch, we gathered for a presentation about the law, this time by a representative from the Karnataka State AIDS Prevention Society (KSAPS), with tight jeans and a gruff tone. "Now, you know what the law is. You're not supposed to send people [facilitate others' sex work]. You have to agree to the law, don't you?" A tall woman in a bright green sari called out, "Well, the law doesn't agree to us either, does it?" The presenter continued, ignoring her. "Now, is the law going to change? No. If you wanted to change it, you'd have to start a *sangha* [association] for that and protest." He moved into an explanation of which aspects of sex work were criminalized and which were not. "It is fine for you to do sex [work]," he said, "just not to cause trouble to society. Now, what do you do if police come? Well, there are ways to get around the law, right?" There was an uncomfortable silence. "I'm not supposed to tell you," he says. "But look. If you are in a sangha, there's a crisis management team. If you call them, a group of people can come and stop it. If you go the police station alone, they will beat you. If twenty women come, you can beat them!"

As the conversation continued, he continued to move back and forth between hinting at ways to circumvent the law and referring to the law with pious reverence. "We have to follow the law. The law is for all Indians. Can we be Indian and not follow the Indian law? No, we can't. If you do wrong, maybe you won't get caught. But will God know what you've done? Yes." Finally, I raised my hand again. "I'm confused," I said. "Are you telling people the law should be changed or that they should follow it?" "It's two things," he said, switching to English for my benefit. "One is changing the law. They would have to start a sangha for that on their own. And one is implementing the law. But changing the law won't happen so easily." Abruptly, he changed the topic to government services for older sex workers. "Do what is right according to the law, and when you get older, the government is ready to help you with a house and a job," he concluded.

The training session revealed the tensions state agencies faced in navigating HIV prevention with a criminalized high-risk group, as well as the key role NGOs and CBOs played in resolving them. The presenter insisted that his audience—a group of brothel madams who break the law by profession—must respect the law, while simultaneously suggesting ways that, through organizations "outside" the state, they might circumvent or even challenge the law. His prevarications revealed the contradictions in the state's regulation of sex work. As both presenters' irritation with our questions suggested, the tensions remained unresolved. And as Chandra's whispered comments to me showed, her CBO played an important role in mediating between this contradictory state response and the realities of gendered power structures sex workers navigated. She was the one who talked to sex workers about how to negotiate condom use or argued with police to let a detained sex worker go. Tolerating the condom demonstration with an air of bemusement, Chandra and the other organizers laughed in the back room.

By holding the event, Chandra's organization was meeting the formal expectations of the state AIDS control program, its main source of funding. Peer educators from high-risk groups, through organizations like Chandra's, did a significant portion of the government's HIV prevention work. But the work Chandra's organization did to challenge police or support sex workers in negotiating with clients was technically outside the state. The funds to support drop-in centers, and the staff who ran them, were channeled through government but, until 2012, largely came from the Gates Foundation and other donors. Their work operated in an exceptional bureaucratic category, apart from the Indian state's core public health concerns. Donors, NGOs, CBOs, global public health institutions, technical support units, trusts, societies, universities—none of the organizations seemed like traditional organs of the state. And yet, together they constituted the Indian state's response to the AIDS epidemic.

This chapter analyzes the Indian state's hybrid response to AIDS. I argue that the Indian AIDS response created multivalent spaces within which the national state, local civil society, and transnational donors became closely imbricated and unusually interdependent. State officials acknowledged that the public health bureaucracy lacked flexibility and reach and was unable to take on the questions of sexuality and criminalization that were needed to stop the crisis. To respond more quickly, they worked through community organizations led by sex workers and sexual minority groups, while insulating themselves from other parts of the state. This creation of hybrid, autonomous spaces within the state bureaucracy built on colonial and postcolonial legacies of containing deviant sexuality. But this chapter also shows that these HIV prevention programs took on a life of their own. Activists, NGOs, and CBOs recognized the state's dependence on them and leveraged it to demand greater control and resources.

Political sociologists help illuminate the realignments of state practice that took place in India's AIDS response. Peter Evans describes the most effective developmental state as both embedded in civil society and autonomous from it.[1] Along with Patrick Heller, he has called the Indian state "accountable, if not responsive."[2] Indian social movements are wide-ranging and experienced in making demands on the state,[3] while the state is not always capable of delivering on those demands. But in the case of AIDS, the state and donors worked together to create exceptional, relatively autonomous hybrid state agencies that operated differently from the rest of the bureaucracy. These pockets within the state, as Erin McDonnell might call them,[4] were both accountable and responsive to activist demands, where other state agencies may not have been. And they had unusual access to global funding and alliances. This hybridity and relative autonomy, reminiscent of what Tianna Paschel calls segmented institutionalization,[5] allowed AIDS agencies to circumvent the inefficiency or sexual conservatism of other state agencies, while leaving those other state agencies relatively unchanged. Unexpectedly, however, the hybrid state spaces of HIV prevention helped catalyze further activism that sometimes made direct demands on the state at large.

These hybrid forms of governance are not unique to AIDS; scholars have noted the Indian state's response to a range of issues, such as domestic violence and women's empowerment, through civil society organizations, activists, and other actors.[6] This chapter builds on this scholarship in two ways. First, it shows that, in the case of AIDS, a logic of sexual containment[7] with colonial roots, and not simply the dynamics of neoliberalization, underpinned and laid the groundwork for later disjunctures within the state. The response to AIDS in India drew on colonial and postcolonial strategies for managing sexual crisis—containing deviant sexuality in order to manage it—exemplified by the Contagious Diseases Acts. In the early stages of the Indian AIDS response, medical authorities reproduced these strategies of containment. They conflated prostitution with AIDS and the racialized and caste-inflected associations of risk and immorality that went with it. But, unexpectedly, this containment paved the way for a tenuous process of incorporation. Sex worker, sexual minority, and transgender groups became crucial to the AIDS response, and, indirectly and conditionally, part of state programs.[8]

Second, the formation of hybrid pockets within the state to circumvent practical limitations was not just the result of bureaucratic ingenuity, as in some accounts.[9] Instead, it resulted from an ongoing process of struggle. NGOs, CBOs, and activist groups pushed for inclusion, sometimes through more collaborative advocacy and policymaking and sometimes through more confrontational critique and protest.[10] The director of one NGO explained how he had been the one to explain the basics of disease prevention every time a new project director was transferred. "We became the knowledge-able ones," he said. "He or she would have no induction . . . [they] would be selling transformers or edible oil one day and suddenly coming to HIV/AIDS." Another activist said he found a pamphlet their NGO had written in critique of AIDS programs displayed on a bookshelf in the office of a state-level AIDS agency. At the same time, the state and donors provided essential resources to NGOs, CBOs, and activist groups—from the money for bus rides, venue rental, and food for meetings to symbolic legitimacy, legal and media training, and a common platform for conflict and reconciliation. Within the interdependent, hybrid space of HIV prevention, where the state began and ended was difficult to pin down. It was this fraught interface, against the backdrop of global crisis, that made India's AIDS response possible.

THE CONTAINMENT OF RISKY SEXUALITY

The Contagious Diseases Acts provided a template for later state responses to sexual crisis aimed at containing and regulating sexual deviance, and, like those later state responses, elicited individual and collective resistance. The Acts subjected registered prostitutes to mandatory weekly venereal disease checks and detainment in lock hospitals if they were found to be infected; unregistered prostitutes could be fined or imprisoned. The historian Ashwini Tambe shows how Indian women in prostitution used a range of strategies to resist detention and coercive medical surveillance.[11] Some four-fifths of women in prostitution in Bombay evaded the mandatory health checks of the

Contagious Diseases Acts by getting married, claiming to be kept women, petitioning the court, bribing officials, covering for each other, or simply leaving the city. There were forms of collective resistance, too. Historian Philippa Levine writes of an 1888 letter describing how "the prostitutes of Calcutta collectively protested to the Viceroy against the use of 'telescopes' in the medical examinations to which they were subjected."[12] And in Madras, the historian Sarah Hodges finds that women not only evaded the lock hospitals by reorganizing their practices but were also able to draw on them strategically as sites of refuge. During the 1876–78 famine, for example, Bangalore lock hospitals filled with women officials categorized as nonprostitutes who applied to be admitted so they could access food and shelter.[13] These accounts suggest that the management of venereal disease was coercive, but incomplete. It was actively resisted, and sometimes it was a contradictory site of resources.

Starting in the late nineteenth century, the acts were gradually undone. In 1888, following a House of Commons resolution, the governor general of India was instructed to dismantle contagious disease legislation.[14] However, the system of lock hospitals, which had existed before the acts, persisted well after 1888, and the techniques of the Contagious Diseases Acts often reappeared when local authorities faced a new spike in venereal disease.[15] In the late nineteenth and early twentieth century, reformers sought to wipe out prostitution altogether.[16] In the 1920s and 1930s, Calcutta, Bombay, Uttar Pradesh, Punjab, and Mysore passed acts that criminalized aspects of prostitution and stipulated the rehabilitation of prostitutes arrested for soliciting.[17] The shifts followed international pressure to fight sex trafficking. For example, the International Convention for the Suppression of the Traffic in Women and Children was passed in 1921 at the League of Nations.[18] By independence in 1947, the lock hospitals had largely been displaced by a focus on ending sex trafficking and later abolishing prostitution.[19]

In 1986, when the first cases of HIV were detected among six women in prostitution in Madras, state medical authorities reverted to techniques of spatial segregation and coercive detention that recalled the Contagious Diseases Acts.[20] As Siddharth Dube wrote, "Forever after in India, AIDS was thought of as a disease of women prostitutes, merely because the first indigenous cases were detected among them."[21] Medical authorities attempted to detain the women. Two of them escaped, but the other four remained in custody.[22] The one woman in prostitution found to be HIV positive in a West Bengal screening was arrested, and released after legal action.[23] *The Lancet* even reported that the ICMR was offering a "monthly salary of £50" to "any HIV-positive prostitute willing to retire from the profession."[24] In May of 1990, 825 prostitutes were reported to have been rescued from brothels in Bombay and returned to Chennai on a train called the Mukti Express (Freedom Express) where they were detained in a prison facility. Activists from ABVA reported that the police cracked down violently when the women demanded food for themselves and their children, and one later committed suicide.[25] In 1994, the government of Maharashtra considered legislation that would brand sex workers with HIV with indelible ink. In 1996, more than four hundred sex workers were arrested and forcibly tested for HIV on the orders of the Mumbai High Court.[26]

These practices of detention and containment were mainly focused on women in prostitution, because experts tended to deny homosexuality in India.[27] But others faced repression too. For example, in 1989, Dominic d'Souza, a gay man, was forcibly quarantined for two months, in what he would later describe as "the most traumatic experience of my life." Police came to his house in the middle of the night to take him to the police station and conduct a forcible physical examination. He did not even know he was HIV-positive until he saw a nurse write "AIDS" on his admission papers. Medical staff often refused to touch him, preferring to question him from the other side of a closed door.[28]

These attempts at containing deviant sexuality were met with protest. D'Souza's case attracted widespread media attention. His village panchayat submitted a written statement and held a silent march demanding his release. His mother filed a writ petition, with the support of the human rights lawyer Anand Grover and the International Health Organization's I. S. Gilada. In 1985 the High Court amended the Goa Public Health Act, under which d'Souza had been detained, and declared the detention of people with HIV and AIDS no longer mandatory.[29] In 1988, public interest litigation led by Shyamala Nataraj resulted in the release of five HIV-positive sex workers in Chennai two years later. Eventually, some eight hundred detained sex workers with HIV were released from detention in Tamil Nadu.[30] The 1989 AIDS Prevention Bill allowed for random, mandatory blood tests of sex workers. The ABVA protested the bill, and it was withdrawn without reaching the status of an act.[31] These activist efforts pushed the state to recalibrate its strategy of violent containment of high-risk groups.

THE RECONFIGURATION OF THE STATE

The containment of deviant sexuality unexpectedly laid the groundwork for the conditional incorporation of high-risk groups into the state agencies devoted to HIV prevention. If sex workers were the source of AIDS, then sex workers could become the key to stopping it.[32] The reconfiguration of the state began in the early 1990s. The first National AIDS Control Programme (NACP I), initiated in 1992, marked a decisive shift from early efforts to detain and forcibly test sex workers. Of the US$113 million in funding for NACP I, 21% was devoted to "promoting public awareness and community support."[33] It created an independent agency, the National AIDS Control Organization (NACO), that was relatively autonomous, administratively and financially, from the rest of the public health bureaucracy and was headed by a high-ranking official.[34] In 2009, a separate Department of AIDS Control gave NACO further autonomy within the Ministry of Health.[35] This relative autonomy protected AIDS programs from bureaucratic backlogs and allowed for innovation and experimentation. NACO was uniquely embedded in local civil society and uniquely well-resourced by global donors. It was also connected to global circuits of AIDS experts. For example, one interviewee recalled a 1997 trip of NACO officials to learn about Thailand's 100% Condom Program with sex workers, which saw prevention in high-risk groups as key to the AIDS response.[36] It was both engaged with activists and autonomous from them, a state agency and yet independent from the rest of the state.

This reconfiguration of the state had several specific benefits for the AIDS response. First, hybrid institutions like NACO could escape the inefficiencies of the public health bureaucracy. They could make decisions, receive and disburse funds, and respond to problems more quickly. Second, state officials had recognized their inability to reach high-risk groups, noting that "socially marginalized sections . . . are not normally accessible through the traditional government machinery."[37] To reach these groups, they increasingly realized, they would have to go outside the usual inflexibility of the bureaucracy. They would have to go to the bus stands, public parks, and red-light districts and take the time to build relationships. Finally, this reconfiguration allowed state agencies to bypass laws and stigma around sexuality. Aspects of both sex work and homosexuality were criminalized, a fact that made official public health outreach difficult. As a semi-independent body, NACO aligned itself with social movements against criminalization but retained a strategic distance.

With this hybrid structure, NACO could work around dominant sexual norms and reach marginalized populations through social movements, even when those social movements targeted the state. In an interview, a NACO official noted,

> Today, for example, in Delhi streets, we find Pride marches take place. . . . those changes come because of not just political interventions or government programs, but the way society responds to some of these things. . . . [Does the state have a role to play?] State has a role to play but we can't leave everything to state. Sometimes state needs to be pressurized through these organized social movements. [So the state has to set up institutions to pressure itself?] Yeah! That is a clever way of doing it. You set up an institution and use that as a pressure group to put pressure on the government. NACO was a state creation, but NACO sometimes becomes an activist organization.

Engaging with activists directly created external pressure on state HIV agencies to respond with urgency. The official continued,

> Activism around AIDS is dying, which is a bad thing. You have to keep the activism alive. . . . Initially there was. I used to face a very aggressive group of activists. Today it doesn't happen. [A lot of the activism was against you!] Initially. To do more. That was a positive thing. At the time I have not taken it in a wrong way. I thought these are the people who have AIDS and are going to die if we don't do something for them. So I engaged with them. [That's not a common thing.] Not very common. Especially among my tribe!

For NACO, then, activist involvement made it possible to address a broader range of social issues, while creating the pressure for the bureaucracy to respond quickly. But it was also important for NACO to retain its independence from activist sex workers, sexual minorities, and transgender people. During an interview with another NACO official, I asked about NACO's position on current policy debates surrounding sex work. He said he could not comment because it was beyond his mandate:

NACO's perspective is protect them from HIV/AIDS. And make sure they are getting care services. That's our only mandate. As an NGO, as a CBO, they can go beyond that, but it's up to them. We make the platform. Suppose they want a social protection scheme. We don't have any provision for giving a social protection scheme. But once they come together, they can approach any organization, any agency, any government agency, they can get it. . . . That is real empowerment. . . . We are not part of any protest. . . . But any organization, they are independent, they can have their own.

For this interviewee, NACO effectively outsourced the challenges to dominant sexual moralities that it could not take on directly. NACO itself could not take a position on sex workers' rights. NGOs and CBOs did that, but they were independent. These independent organizations received funds from NACO and helped write NACO policy. Yet their independence allowed them to mobilize around controversial positions NACO itself could not pursue.

Working through NGOs and CBOs also meant that, in the early years of the AIDS response, these organizations faced the brunt of the violence from other arms of the state and, particularly, the police. A 2002 report from Human Rights Watch, *Epidemic of Abuse,* described a range of incidents of police brutality; in Bangalore, the NGO Samraksha reported twenty incidents of police violence against twenty-seven peer educators and other sex workers, including beating, extortion, sexual assault, and false drug charges; peer educators experienced police throwing their condoms out, taking their bags, destroying their identity cards, and tearing up their educational materials.[38] The office of the NGO Sangama in Bangalore was searched without a warrant.[39] These incidents occurred around the country. When neighbors attacked a house used by the CBO VAMP in Nippani, Karnataka, police refused to take their complaint, saying sex workers were not "normal citizens"; in Lucknow, staff from the NGO Bharosa Trust were imprisoned for forty-seven days.[40] Human Rights Watch recommended that NACO take a public stand in support of the decriminalization of homosexuality and in support of sex workers' rights but quoted NACO officials as saying it was simply a "localized problem" that NGOs should solve by "sensitizing" the police with training.[41] NGOs thus allowed the state to effectively sidestep the violent consequences of HIV prevention.

While depending on their efforts to make HIV prevention possible, the state tended to mark high-risk groups as outside of the normal workings of government. Sex workers, sexual minorities, and transgender people were not part of the state machinery. They were conditionally included,[42] needed mainly to stem the greater threat of HIV reaching the general population. NACO documents noted, "When the community defines HIV prevention as part of its own agenda, uptake of services and commodities is higher than when services are 'imposed' upon it."[43] Government officials, NACP III documents pointed out, could never have "as full or the same picture as HRGs themselves,"[44] and if high-risk groups themselves drove the response, they could then play the role of a "pressure group" as consumers to push for higher quality services.[45] The long-term aim of NACP III was for prevention programs to be run completely by community members, "thereby putting the prevention responsibility on those who are themselves at risk."[46]

While state AIDS officials distanced themselves from community-based organizations when it came to challenging the criminalization of deviant sexuality, in other ways they celebrated their successes and their global acclaim. One state-level AIDS official described a successful local sex worker organization: "They developed the concept of empowerment of sex workers. This is an international event. No country in the world has developed this model. They started the intervention . . . to protect health, and after that came empowerment, rights, and other things. . . . They have shown the path of how to empower sex workers through awareness . . . not just themselves but with local stakeholders and powerholders in society." When I asked what the state's role had been in this international event, he insisted that its role was mainly auxiliary. "SACS [State AIDS Control Societies] provides necessary financial and logistical support. . . . There is no such empowerment model within SACS. We supported as a state body and mentor [CBOs] as per national policy." The words *support* and *mentor* appeared often in my interviews with government officials when it came to their role in HIV prevention with high-risk groups. The state's role was mainly financial and logistical, and it relied on community-based organizations to engage in the necessary work of empowerment that it could not (or would not) do on its own.

As this interviewee's references to global acclaim suggest, the global AIDS field played an important role in laying the institutional groundwork for the insulation of HIV prevention from the rest of the public health bureaucracy, both in terms of symbolic and material resources. A key donor in the early years was the World Bank.[47] The World Bank contributed a US$84 million credit to the NACP I effort, making the AIDS response uniquely well-funded compared to other disease control efforts. The Bank's influence was not only financial but also political. A NACO official at the time explained in an interview, "If the Bank guy comes and tells something to the political leaders here, they listen." The Bank shaped the direction of the AIDS response in line with neoliberal governance mechanisms popular at the time: hybrid public-private institutions, devolution of control to the local level, and participation from civil society.[48] The Bank pushed for a role for NGOs in the AIDS response, while training NGOs to implement programs according to donor directives.[49]

As AIDS programs gained momentum and resources in their second round, NACP II, donor involvement expanded and diversified. The World Bank continued to play a role in policy formulation, but as NACO established a reputation, it attracted a wider range of donors. Thus, in 1999, the budget for national AIDS control quadrupled to US$460 million,[50] with the Bank contributing $242 million and a variety of donors contributing the rest, including a substantial $102 million from the British DfID and $35 million from USAID.[51] In 2003, the Gates Foundation's Avahan program was launched, committing $258 million until 2008 for its six focus states, Andhra Pradesh, Karnataka, Maharashtra, Manipur, Nagaland, and Tamil Nadu.[52] With its greater funding and technical expertise, NACO also began to set its own priorities, asking donors to, according to one former NACO director, "put the money into the kitty" so that it could decide where to direct resources and how to prioritize programs. A NACO official noted in an interview,

> We were firm on that. I thought that if these people are allowed to go and let loose, then they will choose programs which will appeal to them. And then they will start funding, and when the donor starts funding, they will put a lot of money into management, they will have high salaries, you know, to managers, high salaries to peer educators, so you basically create something like an island of affluence, among others who get money from the government. . . . Whereas government programs are sustainable over a long period of time, because there is government commitment to the people, the donor is there so long as their money lasts, and after that they leave.

NACO thus maintained autonomy not only from other parts of the state but also from donors. There was a major spike in AIDS funding as India became known as the next epicenter of the epidemic. In the third round of the National AIDS Control Programme, NACP III, the budget again more than quadrupled to $2.5 billion. India's receipt of foreign funds for AIDS peaked in 2007–2008 in the period between 1999 and 2012: the Organisation for Economic Co-operation and Development (OECD) reported that donors committed $787 million in aid to India for STDs and AIDS in 2007. AIDS funding accounted for nearly 10% of all foreign contributions to Indian associations and organizations in the 2008–2009 financial year.[53] In 2008, the Gates Foundation pledged an additional $80 million, to be used before 2013. NACO reported that about 60% of funds for NACP III came from external assistance.[54]

The relatively autonomous and hybrid structure of NACO extended to state-level agencies, which were also globally funded and intimately engaged with civil society. Under NACP I, NACO created SACS in each state that reported to NACO. The SACS were registered as societies rather than treated as government departments, which allowed them to avoid the backlogs in fund disbursal that often plagued government agencies. Once the Gates Foundation's Avahan program came into the picture in 2003, additional partnerships were formed. In Karnataka, the Karnataka Health Promotion Trust (KHPT) was jointly managed by KSAPS and the University of Manitoba, and it served as the state lead partner for the Avahan program. This hybrid structure meant KHPT was less bound by government norms and thus quicker to act. One official noted, "With government, we lacked timely access to funds. They [government] are answerable. Their policies are guided by the Constitution. Government norms are broader, less flexible. KHPT was more flexible, and could make quicker decisions."

By the mid-2000s, the AIDS response was increasingly separate from the rest of the public health system. NACO's exceptional status within the Ministry of Health and Family Welfare, with its network of state AIDS control organizations registered as societies, managing donor funds in partnership with NGOs, separated AIDS control from governance as usual.

LAW, SEXUALITY, AND CONFLICTS WITHIN THE STATE
The hybrid spaces within the state devoted to HIV prevention—uniquely engaged with sex worker, sexual minority, and transgender activists and

NGOs—put NACO at odds with other state agencies. The Immoral Traffic (Prevention) Act treated largely conflated prostitution with sex trafficking and effectively criminalized it; under the Indian Penal Code, homosexuality was criminalized. "On one side they give us condoms; on the other side they arrest us," observed a sex worker I met in Maharashtra through the activist group VAMP. A UN researcher whom I interviewed described this split in the government as "schizophrenic." Ravi, a government official employed at the state level in Karnataka, observed,

> NACO knows the issues of these communities. . . . in government it's like actually one part of government knows something about some issues, and one part of government knows it differently. . . . So if a person [uses] heroin, we [NACO] will give a new needle, but if a police officer finds him, he will arrest him. So it's the same government, but we know these are different, and HIV I think has brought a new perspective to government itself. . . . compared to the other departments, I think [this is] the first time the government is working with community in a large way. . . . I don't think any other [government] department in India is working with such a close relationship with the community that they are addressing. . . . So it's the first time, I think, because of HIV, the national government is also interested in communities. [The government needed the community.] Yeah. The government needed the community because it's, it's not only a medical problem, it's a behavioral issue, so to change their behavior you have to have them on board.

Ravi pointed out that NACO was uniquely engaged with communities at risk of HIV.[55] Because of the exceptional nature of HIV prevention, community participation was necessary to stem the epidemic. This engagement, he pointed out, made NACO unique among state agencies. Thus, within the same state apparatus, the same problem could be understood and managed in vastly different ways, and NACO was more embedded in civil society than other state agencies.

Not only was NACO unique among state agencies, other interviewees echoed, it was also unique among public health programs. One NACO official I interviewed noted that "other disease control programmes" were "less participatory, more centralized and prescriptive, rigid, and tend more to biomedical than social dimensions." A UN researcher pointed out that this engagement with civil society, tied to a human rights perspective, was also true of the global AIDS field:

> HIV has really been basically an entry point for taking a human rights approach to all kinds of things. It really is fascinating. HIV is an entry point for human rights programming. Any kind of human rights programming. That distinguishes our approaches to HIV from our approach to leprosy, tuberculosis, malaria, or whatever other disease. Our approach to other diseases has not been about human rights approaches. With tuberculosis, 40–60 years ago, and even 5 years ago, outside of the HIV context, nobody was really saying that in addressing TB we absolutely must look at poverty or the human rights of those people. That was not where medicine went at all. HIV almost solely has started a human rights approach.

HIV prevention, then, as these interviewees pointed out, moved away from traditional biomedical approaches to more rights-based approaches. As NACO's structure grew more complex, and its engagement with community organizations deepened, it broadened its focus beyond the traditional realm of public health. NACP II argued that "HIV/AIDS is not merely a public health challenge, it is also a political and social challenge" and called for a "paradigm shift" toward "a more holistic approach looking at AIDS as a developmental problem.[56] The NACP III development process involved more collaboration with nongovernmental entities than ever before, with fourteen working groups, composed of experts and activists from NGOs and CBOs, conducting consultations all over the country.[57] Nearly 70% of the NACP III budget was earmarked for prevention efforts, a third of which was to go to high-risk groups.[58] The policy now explicitly included attention to "the enabling environment" for high-risk groups—the legal and political context that shaped these groups' ability to practice safer sex—addressing "key stakeholders" and "power structures," "crisis management systems," and "legal rights."[59] NACP IV argued that "people fighting the battle with or of HIV/AIDS are valued citizens, whose life is as important as anyone else's."[60]

As NACO broadened its engagement with sexual minority groups and sex workers, its conflict with other state agencies grew more pronounced. Laws around sexuality proved to be a flash point. In 2006, the Ministry of Women and Child Development proposed a set of amendments to the

ITPA, the Immoral Traffic (Prevention) Act. ITPA had changed little since its first passage in 1956, except to become gender-neutral. It did not technically prohibit the act of prostitution, but it did give police officers and local magistrates considerable power to harass and detain sex workers indefinitely for related offenses, like soliciting or living off the earnings of a prostitute.[61] The ITPA was thus at odds with an HIV prevention strategy that employed and collaborated with sex workers to conduct peer health outreach. The new amendments criminalized clients of sex workers. The proposal proved to be a galvanizing force for sex worker organizations around the country, and sex workers attended rallies, wrote letters, and participated in consultations demanding the proposal be rejected. They argued that the proposal would drive sex work underground, hurting their livelihoods as well as HIV prevention efforts. NACO itself submitted statements against the amendments, pitting two governmental agencies against each other.[62] The New Delhi–based NGO Lawyer's Collective issued a statement that the amendments would "undermine HIV prevention, increase transmission and endanger the health of millions in this country."[63] Eventually, the bill was suspended, and sex worker activists considered their efforts a success. "Our best support was HIV," said an interviewee at the Lawyer's Collective. "The message was very clear: if you criminalize clients, all your interventions will collapse."[64] At the same time, she noted, state responsiveness to sex workers' experience of criminalization was conditional and partial: "India's managed to contain HIV without reforming sex work law." Researchers from the Durbar Mahila Samanwaya Committee and VAMP have continued to document the devastating effects of police raids on sex workers.[65]

AIDS also became an important catalyst in the struggle to decriminalize homosexuality. After recommending that condoms be provided to men in prisons and being refused on the grounds that homosexuality was illegal in India, the ABVA filed the first petition challenging the constitutional validity of anti-sodomy law (Section 377 of the Indian Penal Code) in the Delhi High Court in 1994.[66] Seven years later, the Naz Foundation filed public interest litigation seeking repeal of Section 377. In 2009, the Delhi High Court overturned Section 377, effectively rendering homosexuality legal. NACO submitted an affidavit in support of overturning Section 377, arguing that it hampered HIV prevention efforts and thus obstructed the right to health.[67] Activists I interviewed agreed that AIDS arguments played a key role in their arguments for decriminalizing homosexuality, even as they limited the scope of human rights claims.[68] NACO's engagement with civil society facilitated challenges to laws that hindered HIV prevention. It thus circumvented sexual norms and legal structures that would have otherwise taken much longer to shift, and it supported gains for the LGBTQIA+ movement at the same time.

THE GOVERNMENT IS DEPENDENT ON US

NACO's hybrid structure and engagement with community organizations was not just the result of an ideological commitment nor was it an enlightened strategy for efficient crisis response. It was not predetermined or preplanned. Instead, it was an uneven response to both donor pressure and the demands for participation from groups of sex workers, sexual minorities, and transgender people with growing global support. Activists, NGOs, and CBOs demanded a role not just in implementing HIV prevention programs but also in planning and conceptualizing them. These demands came from a key recognition: the government was dependent on sex workers, sexual minorities, and transgender people for its interventions to function. One NGO worker explained,

> After HIV came . . . [the government] are all doing this for sex workers, not because we love sex workers. . . . They are less than one percent of the population. . . . I can't distribute condoms to 99% of people, my public health approach, my expenditure, will not allow me to do [so]. . . . It is easy for me to distribute condoms to 1% and keep them safe. Why am I keeping them safe? Not because I love them. I love this 99%. . . . This for the first few years, sex workers didn't know. Slowly they started learning this fact. Government is not doing it for our sake. We are the pillars of the prevention. We are at the forefront. Unless we do [our work], NGO can't do anything, government can't do anything. Once that feeling, that realization came, once NGOs also realized it, sex workers started empowering themselves. . . . That brought a big change in the sex workers' movement.

This interviewee underscored the role of sex workers' own demands in leveraging the state's strategy of containing risk into a demand for incorporation. I heard this acknowledgment several times from sex worker, sexual minority, and transgender organizers during my fieldwork. As one outreach worker and transgender woman sex worker put it, "It's because of us that [NGOs] get those HIV funds. Without us, they'd be nothing."[69] The continued participation of sex workers, sexual minorities, and transgender people and their willingness to be tested, documented, and surveyed about their sexual lives were central to the success of HIV prevention programs. Donors and the state depended on NGOs, who in turn depended on CBOs, who in turn depended on their members, to contain HIV risk. This chain of dependence meant a certain leverage to challenge the rules.

An early step toward demanding incorporation was pushing middle-class allies to think holistically about AIDS. Many of the prominent activist allies I interviewed described moments when they had been forced to reconsider their preconceptions about sexuality and rethink their approach to HIV prevention. Shyamala Nataraj, for example, who led the first activist efforts in Chennai in the 1980s, described an encounter at a vigilance home where HIV-positive sex workers had been forcibly detained:

> And [the superintendent] said, you know, this lady's come, she has a lot of money, she's going to come and help you. . . . Then one girl, she couldn't have been older than you, probably younger, very beautiful, came up to me and sort of spat on my face. And she said you come here, you write about us, you make money, you publish these things, you have a name, while we continue to stay like this. What right do you have? Who gives you the right to come and do this? It's because I'm poor, and you're rich. . . . They say I have AIDS. So what? My parents will take care of me. Who are you to tell me that I can't be with them? Then she said if you come back one more time, I'll kill you and then I'll kill myself. And she turned around and ran off, just sobbing, and a lot of women followed her.[70]

The scene Nataraj paints here is one of a moment of reckoning in which she was forced to reconsider what she thought she knew. Another NGO director I interviewed recalled how she had come to notice the insufficiency of narrow biomedical approaches to HIV prevention: "We felt that everybody's talking about the infection and the public health part of it, but very few people are talking about the individuals involved. . . . And actually what are their needs? . . . . So even our first program with women in sex work was called sex worker protection program. Not HIV prevention program." Being exposed to the experiences of sex workers had pushed Chitra to focus her activism beyond the ambit of existing HIV prevention programs to focus on the social and emotional needs of sex workers.

The formation of several pioneering organizations working with sex workers, sexual minorities, and transgender people on HIV prevention in the 1980s and 1990s laid the groundwork for their later involvement in national AIDS programs. Many developed a prominent presence before they became involved in government programs and, indeed, before the government began to take working with high-risk groups seriously. In the 1990s, several key organizations formed: South India AIDS Action Project in Chennai in 1991;[71] Sampada Grameen Mahila Sanstha (SANGRAM) in Sangli, Maharashtra in 1992; Y.R. Gaitonde Centre for AIDS Research and Education in Chennai, Belgaum Integrated Rural Development Society (BIRDS) in Belgaum,[72] and Samraksha in Bangalore all in 1993; the Naz Foundation in Delhi and Humsafar Trust in Mumbai both in 1994; and Sangama in Bangalore in 1999. In the mid-2000s, as Gates Foundation funding helped scale up HIV prevention efforts, additional NGOs formed that would become important players in HIV prevention programs nationally, including Swasti in Bangalore in 2002 and Ashodaya Samithi in Mysore in 2003. These organizations bolstered their efforts to demand incorporation into AIDS programs by emphasizing to the state and donors their efficacy at HIV prevention while pushing to broaden biomedical efforts into more social and political goals.

One key example of this broadening of HIV prevention goals was the Durbar Mahila Samanwaya Committee, or "Unstoppable Women's Coordinating Committee" (DMSC), a collective of sixty-five thousand sex workers first established in the Sonagachi district of Kolkata in West Bengal.[73] My interviewees generally agreed that it was a pioneer in sex worker mobilization. "Once DMSC started, then the mobilization process started in India," said one AIDS researcher. DMSC began as a public health program. In 1992, just as NACP I began to take shape, the All India Institute of Hygiene and Public Health in Kolkata, along with an NGO called the Society for Community Development, conducted a baseline study of sex workers' practices, condom use, and STD and HIV prevalence in Sonagachi, Kolkata's oldest and most well-known red-light district.[74] Following the initial study, the institute recruited Smarajit Jana, an epidemiologist then working as an assistant professor of occupational health, to initiate an STD/HIV Intervention Project among sex workers in Kolkata. Described by its architects as "unplanned and atheoretical,"[75] the project began with a peer education model, hiring sex workers to distribute condoms and talk about STI and HIV prevention in the brothels in the red-light district. Over time, the project gradually took on environmental components that were shaping sex workers' ability to use condoms, such as violence and extortion from the police or discrimination against sex workers by health professionals.

What became known as the Sonagachi model began from the idea of sex work as work and HIV as an occupational hazard. In 1995, the DMSC formed as a sex-worker–led collective that began expanding its work to red-light districts outside of Sonagachi, taking on police repression and eviction by holding rallies and contesting arrests, as well as building links to other sex worker organizations around the country. DMSC's manifesto at the 1997 National Sex Workers' Conference presented a challenge to narrow conceptions of sex workers within the AIDS policies that had first inspired its formation. "Even to realise the very basic Project objectives of controlling transmission of HIV and STD it was crucial to view us in our totality," it argued, "as complete persons with a range of emotional and material needs, living within a concrete and specific social, political and ideological context which determine the quality of our lives and our health, and not see us merely in terms of our sexual behavior."[76] DMSC's manifesto directly took on both issues of class and work and issues of sexual repression, asking questions like, "What is the history of sexual morality? Why have we circumscribed sexuality within such a narrow confine, ignoring its many other expressions, experiences, and manifestations?" and "Do men and women have equal claims to sexuality?" The manifesto began with the line, "A new spectre seems to be haunting the society." It explained how sex work fit into broader patterns of poverty and unemployment in India and called for an end to sexual moralities that stigmatized sex workers.[77]

As DMSC grew in influence and scope, it took on a variety of issues. Activists consciously identified trade unionism as an inspiration. DMSC operates a cooperative society that provides loans and savings to sex workers, with nearly twenty thousand members and a turnover of over US$2 million. Initially funded by British DfID and later by NACO, it receives funding from the WHO as well as members who give the organization 2% of their salary. DMSC developed an activist political culture.[78] The organization includes several linked organizations, including one of sex workers' children and one of sex workers' partners. In 2010, DMSC began working to organize domestic workers and construction workers with funding from Tata Trust, a private philanthropic organization. It also set up self-regulatory boards as an alternative to policing in the red-light districts. "We have no interest in HIV now," said a DMSC leader in an interview. "We've moved from HIV to being a big union." DMSC was often called on to represent sex workers on national and international consultations.[79]

Another key organization that gained global and national prominence was SANGRAM. According to my interviews, SANGRAM had first been registered in 1986 as a women's organization but had since become defunct. In 1992, Meena Seshu began identifying peer educators for an HIV prevention initiative in Gokulnagar, a red-light area in Sangli, Maharashtra, and revived the organization.[80] SANGRAM grew into a "series of collective empowerment groups for stigmatized communities" in southern Maharashtra and northern Karnataka.[81] The collectives under the SANGRAM umbrella include Veshya Anyay Mukti Parishad, a group of five thousand women in sex work, formed in 1996; Muskan, a collective of male and trans sex workers, formed in 2000; and Mitra, a collective of children of sex workers, formally established in 2009. SANGRAM also supports a collective of rural women workers, called Vidrohi Mahila Manch; one of Muslim women, called Nazariya; and one of HIV-positive women, called SANGRAM Plus.[82] It has facilitated several key research projects, such as the Pan-India Survey of Sex Workers[83] and, more recently, a study of the effects of anti-trafficking raids.[84]

Seshu's background in the feminist movement led her to approach HIV prevention from the perspective of sex workers' self-determination rather than what she considered the more instrumental approach of containing deviant sexuality and focusing solely on condom use.[85] While she began with a focus on rescue, she learned to "listen to women" and think about sex work as "for these women to make money."[86] In reclaiming terms like *veshya* [prostitute] and Indian histories of sexual service provision, SAN-GRAM today urges a rejection of "white colonial" conceptions of "selling sex." A 1998 *Statement of Women in Prostitution* offered a distinctly feminist perspective on sex work. It argued that "prostitution is a way of life like any other," not a long-term profession but a transient occupation among others, and pointed out that, while "all occupations stereotypical to women adhere to so-called 'feminine values,'" and prostitution was in this way similar to being a housewife, a nurse, or a receptionist, women in prostitution enjoyed economic independence and were "more empowered than most women within male-dominated patriarchal structures." The statement argued that "a woman's sexuality is an integral part of her as a woman" and challenged the stigmatization of sex work, while also protesting "a society that aggressively promotes objectification and commercialization of women and their sexuality" and "globalization and economic liberalization."[87] The statement articulated a feminist conceptualization of sex workers' rights entirely distinct from the needs of HIV prevention; indeed, HIV and AIDS were not even mentioned.

Organizations like DMSC and SANGRAM gained influence on the state in part through the global acclaim they quickly garnered for their work. Their relationships with Amnesty International, UNFPA, the Open Society Foundation, UNAIDS, and Hivos demonstrated an ability to align with the global AIDS field and win global support. UNAIDS hailed the Sonagachi Project for its "integral involvement of sex workers" and its demonstration that "even in highly repressive and abusive environments, the rights of sex workers can be addressed and sex workers themselves can be enabled to act."[88] A widely cited UNAIDS report argued that the Sonagachi Project was "one of the most sustainable, if not biomedically perfect, in the reality of an imperfect world."[89] In the 2006 *Report on the Global AIDS Epidemic*, UNAIDS mentioned sex workers as "among the most effective actors in HIV responses" and Sonagachi as "a touchstone for sex worker projects around the world."[90] SANGRAM gained support from a variety of donors, including the Ford Foundation and the American Jewish World Service. It was even able to challenge global donors' approaches to sex work. In 2003, for example, funding from the Avert Society, a joint project of NACO, the Government of India, and USAID, through the Bush-era US President's Emergency Plan for AIDS Relief, required what is typically called the *anti-prostitution pledge*, in line with the US government's policy that funds could not go to an organization without "a policy explicitly opposing prostitution and sex trafficking."[91] SANGRAM turned down the US$20,000 in funds, arguing that "we are not traffickers; simply a sex workers' collective wanting recognition of our rights."[92]

Sex worker organizations in India evolved alongside and helped to create broader shifts in the politics of sex work within the UN and other global institutions. Priscilla Alexander, a founding member of Call Off Your Old Tired Ethics (COYOTE), a sex worker activist group in San Francisco, and the founder of the California Prostitutes Education Project, became a consultant to the WHO's Global Programme on AIDS in 1989. She helped lay the foundation for the WHO and other global public health institutions to engage with rights-based HIV prevention for sex workers. In a 2008 address to the International AIDS Conference, Ban Ki-Moon argued that "in countries without laws to protect sex workers, drug users, and men who have sex with men, only a fraction of the population has access to prevention. . . . Not only is it unethical not to protect these groups, it makes no sense from a health perspective. It hurts all of us."[93]

Indian organizations were a key voice in shifts in the global AIDS field surrounding sex workers' rights and contributed to several important debates. Between 2007 and 2009, the Global Working Group on HIV and Sex Work Policy rewrote the controversial *UNAIDS Guidance Note on HIV and Sex Work*, citing SANGRAM and DMSC as examples of good practice.[94] It was ultimately India's National Network of Sex Workers that presented the new draft to UNAIDS.[95] SANGRAM has made formal submissions to international treaty bodies and UN agencies, such as the Convention on the Elimination of All Forms of Discrimination against Women and the Special Rapporteur on Violence against Women, as well as, at the national level, to panels such as the Justice Verma Committee, which made recommendations on laws relating to sexual assault in India.[96] In my interviews, local government officials often referred admiringly to the global recognition sex worker organizations received. These growing alignments with the global field heightened activists' ability to influence local and national AIDS programs.

CONFLICT AND INTERDEPENDENCE

The expansive work of organizations like DMSC and SANGRAM, and their alignments with the global field, helped advance their role in shaping hybrid pockets of the state devoted to HIV prevention. In Bangalore, the relationship between the state and sex workers, sexual minorities, and transgender people was variable. Some organizations were dependent on the state and donors for conceptual direction, some more collaborative, and some more oppositional. Yet interviewees from a range of organizations noted the uniquely hybrid, relatively autonomous nature of AIDS agencies and the opening for participation it provided. One activist noted, for example, their ability to influence KHPT, the state-university held trust that managed Gates Foundation funds in Karnataka:

> We don't see KHPT as government—government is the ministries, etc. We deal with those like any other movement does. . . . KHPT is nothing. [They are] scared of us, you know, they know that we can protest and shut down their office anytime . . . and they also know that we can go to the health minister and get them into trouble. That fear is always there when they negotiate with us. Also somewhere I think the bureaucrats . . . they treat us better, because they know that we are powerful. Even though we disagree with them, they have respect for us. Others, who are their puppets, they don't respect them.

Another activist noted, "Now the government is dependent on [us.] [Why?] Because we are close to sex workers and sexual minorities." She added that organizations that could be relied on to do the job effectively were particularly valuable to state agencies desperate to reach marginalized groups but with little understanding of how to do so.

Some NGOs saw their relationship to the state as collaborative. One NGO director argued that "the government is controlling many things," but "development is far too complex for one person" and should ultimately involve "private, government, NGO all put together." For other organizations, the dynamic was more of a push-and-pull relationship of conflict and negotiation, what Chaitanya Lakkimsetti calls a pragmatic approach.[97] One NGO director explained,

> We were definitely one of KHPT's best partners. Without a doubt. Then we got them and we started challenging them . . . [How open were they to pushing the boundaries of what they thought you should be doing?] It was a very mixed bag. Sometimes they were supportive, sometimes they were not, sometimes they thought we were being too unreasonable, sometimes we felt they were being unreasonable. But it was a relationship with a lot of pushes on both sides. They were trying to push, we were trying to push. Sometimes it was very friendly and amicable and agreeable. Sometimes there were things that we didn't do well enough, sometimes there were things that they tried to push which were not OK by us.

Within this push-and-pull relationship, it was clear that activists did benefit from the platform and funding AIDS programs provided. AIDS provided unique pathways to influence for sex workers and sexual minority groups. Community organizations and activists recognized the unique moment of dependence the global pressure to respond to HIV had created. This recognition gave them unprecedented room to challenge state agencies and demand greater inclusion in decision-making processes. The state needed activists to stop AIDS, and activists wanted the state to recognize the immediate needs of sex workers, sexual minorities, and transgender people.

A protest in Bangalore in the fall of 2012 demonstrated the intimate and fraught relationship between the state and the high-risk groups it needed to engage to stop AIDS. The morning of the protest, sex worker, sexual minority, transgender activists, and CBO workers arrived from all over the state to demand higher wages for the HIV prevention work they did. We sat in a circle of plastic chairs preparing to protest. "There's NACO, and below that KSAPS [the Karnataka State AIDS Prevention Society], and below that the ORWs [outreach workers working for NGOs and CBOs], and below that the peers [peer educators working for NGOs and CBOs]," said one of the activists in a rousing tone. "Who's at the bottom?" "The peers," everyone called out. "Who does all the work?" "The peers," we all responded. "Who do we protest?" he went on. "The government," everyone responded. "But," he pointed out, "CBOs can't protest the government because they get money from the government. So in every district there should be somebody that can protest." The protest was organized by a group of NGO and CBO workers and activists, protesting state exploitation as an independent body. After lunch, buses took people to Bangalore's Town Hall. The group crowded on the steps of the building to chant together. "We are not volunteers, we are workers!" "No to unjust targets!" and "Down with NACO!" The protest made clear that the boundaries of the state were contested and porous. Many of the protestors were paid stipends through government mechanisms and had organized for the protest through government-funded CBOs, but they were nevertheless marked as outside the typical workings of the state. In demanding recognition as government workers, they leveraged their conditional inclusion in HIV programs to demand status as state employees.

In everyday life, too, associations with government gave sex workers, sexual minorities, and transgender people a certain sense of legitimacy.

During my fieldwork, peer educators regularly referred to their programs as dependent on government money and their incomes as government pay. They also talked about the emotional impact of being acknowledged and recognized by the government through HIV prevention programs. Once, I walked home with Amitha, an elected leader at a sex worker CBO, to conduct an interview. I soon realized that it would be impossible to conduct the interview as I normally did because Amitha's son and mother-in-law, who did not know she did sex work, were both sitting in the room. We talked in a kind of doublespeak, discussing her organizational role without ever actually naming her work. I began asking more generic questions about her work at the CBO, until her mother-in-law, now bursting with curiosity, asked what the organization did. "It's government, Amma [mother]," she said. "The organization is just like the central government. They go to foreign countries and everything. Big people come."

Amitha was not simply enchanted by an image of state protection or aspiring to the state as a benefactor.[98] Rather, she was leveraging her association with the state strategically to navigate her family's questions.[99] Conversations like the one I had in Amitha's house happened over and over in my fieldwork. I learned to talk about sex work and sexuality without talking about it, to use code words and lowered breath, and to talk about HIV in order to avoid talking about sex. I also learned that invoking the government was an easy way to lend seriousness and respectability to HIV prevention work. Most of my interviewees told me their families knew they did social work or worked for the government but not what they did or why they did it. Association with the state, and with the urgent work of disease prevention, gave organizing sex workers, sexual minorities, and transgender people a practical moral legitimacy. In her own way, Amitha had drawn on her organization's association with the government and with global donors to bolster the legitimacy of her work. Paradoxically, she was criminalized by the very state that depended on her, and she had leveraged that dependence to stake a claim.

REIMAGINING THE STATE

Outside of HIV prevention spaces, for sex worker, sexual minority, and transgender groups, the state held a complex mix of disappointments and fears.[100] "They're not even looking in our direction," said Sudha, a transgender woman. For others, encounters with the state had mainly been encounters

GIVES RESPECTABILITY TO SEX WORKERS

with the police. Chandrakant, a bisexual man, told me, "The government has not done anything good. They use the law to make things difficult for us. They say [homosexuality] is illegal. They keep an eye on people like us, follow their activities, catch them in the courts, and fill them with fear." I often heard accounts of violence and corruption in encounters with the police, alongside accounts of sex and flirtation,[101] alongside accounts of state neglect. As Sudha and Chandrakant's opposing accounts illustrate, my interviewees imagined the state as simultaneously ubiquitous and remote, powerful and dependent, protective and predatory, and dangerous and desirable.

The response to the AIDS crisis reconfigured the Indian state's regulation of sexuality, creating hybrid spaces of access and negotiation. Sex work and homosexuality were accepted, even cautiously affirmed, within AIDS agencies, though they continued to be criminalized by other parts of the state. Within these AIDS spaces, sex workers, sexual minorities, and transgender people received their salaries from government funds for implementing a government program. They were a central feature of a government effort that had won global acclaim. Once punished and detained for spreading AIDS, they were now the forefront of the AIDS response. This shift from containment to incorporation unfolded through a process of struggle. State officials recognized their own limitations, while sex worker, sexual minority, and transgender groups increasingly organized at the local and national level, demanded further involvement in decision making. On both sides, alignments with the global AIDS field played a crucial role. Donors pumped resources into the Indian AIDS response and insisted on its autonomy from other areas of public health. And sex worker, sexual minority, and transgender organizations drew material and symbolic support from global institutions. This global alignment strengthened their demands on the state.

The disjunctures within the Indian state as it responded to the AIDS crisis align with the work of scholars who argue that the boundaries between state and civil society grow increasingly porous with the advance of neoliberalization.[102] Yet the ongoing struggle of sex worker, sexual minority, and transgender activists to resist their containment to the pockets to which they had been relegated suggest that the boundaries of state and society are not endlessly blurred.[103] This chapter has charted their tenuous relationship of interdependence and conflict in the spaces of HIV prevention.[104] For state officials, managing AIDS through community organizations was a way to displace responsibility for HIV prevention. Containment, after all, is less about protecting those who are contained than it is about protecting the general population. For sex worker, sexual minority, and transgender activists, making demands on the state was a way of countering this logic of sexual containment, of "refusing to let the promise of state protection fade away."[105]

HIV prevention programs paved the way for those defined as high-risk groups to make demands on the state as part of newly energized social movements. The contours of these demands, and the tactics activists used for making them, took on a wide range of articulations and were not limited to seeking leadership within the AIDS response. Sex worker, sexual minority, and transgender groups formed in the context of the AIDS crisis fought to free themselves from their association with AIDS, while leveraging the resources their centrality to the AIDS response generated. In doing so, they drew on alliances within their local political context. In the next chapter I turn to the kinds of claims sex worker organizations made in the context of HIV prevention funding in Bangalore and the various ways in which they drew on local political alliances to transform their designation as at-risk targets of HIV prevention into claims as citizens.

4 | AT-RISK CITIZENS

ON A DRIZZLING AFTERNOON in August 2012, I arrived at Bangalore's Freedom Park for a rally organized by the Pension Parishad. In addition to demanding a universal old-age pension, the Pension Parishad demanded a lower pension eligibility age of fifty for women and forty-five for "highly vulnerable groups," including the "elderly, Dalits, tribal people, marginal farmers, domestic workers, sex workers, transgenders, construction workers and people living with HIV."[1] A stage had been positioned at one end of the large fairground, filled with blue plastic chairs, still mostly empty. Vendors sold water and plastic cups of cut fruit.

In the span of a few minutes, I saw a range of different sex worker groups arrive in the park. Lata arrived at the protest at the front of a large march from another park in the city, holding up a banner for the Pension Parishad, shouting slogans like "*bhikshe beda*, pension *beku*" [We don't want charity, we want a pension]. She was surrounded by fellow sex worker, sexual minority, and transgender activists, many cheering, dancing, and clapping their hands at the front of the procession. A large banner in front clearly identified the group as a union of sex workers, and the mix of transgender women, cisgender women, and kothi protesters highlighted the group's visible transgression of gendered and sexual norms. Then another set of cisgender women went to the stage. Their faces solemn as they gathered around the microphone, they sang a moving song in Kannada, detailing the travails of women in poverty. That they, too, were an organization of sex workers would not have been clear to anyone not familiar with their work. As the rain gathered force, I noticed that there were other organizations of sex workers there too, including one large contingent that had arrived on the bus from Mysore.

The sex worker groups I encountered at the protest were all involved in the AIDS response. However, at this protest, they were not articulating demands in relation to AIDS institutions. Instead, they were making demands for citizenship that aligned them with a broader set of movements of marginalized people. They were engaging the state not as targets of HIV prevention, whose relevance to the nation depended on their high-risk categorization, but as citizens with a legitimate claim on social services.[2] In the 1990s, as Chapter 3 showed, sex worker, sexual minority, and transgender groups gradually became leaders within the AIDS response. By the 2000s and 2010s, these groups were simultaneously making diverse claims on the state that addressed social marginalization, criminalization, and economic exclusion. These groups focused not only on the urgency of the AIDS crisis but also on the enduring everyday crises that shaped their lives.

When I interviewed state officials about AIDS programs, they usually described sex workers or men who have sex with men as a broadly undifferentiated mass, subsumed under the ambiguous word community.[3] The assumed unity was understandable. Several of the organizations at the protest had formed in the last fifteen years, and AIDS programs were a significant source of their financial and institutional support, whether directly or indirectly. Yet there was a wide range of political articulations that emerged within the AIDS response. This chapter argues that sex worker groups articulated citizenship not just in relation to the global AIDS field but also in relation to the varied local landscape of NGOs and social movements.

Theories of articulation, as Stuart Hall puts it, ask "how an ideology discovers its subject."[4] Hall argues that elements of discourse can be articulated in different ideological formations; they have no predetermined unity. Thus, religion, class, or the meanings of blackness can be articulated differently in different contexts. They are related to social conditions but are never inevitable, and they can be transformed in a variety of ways.[5] Hall's conception of articulation offers a flexible, nondeterministic approach to how

TWO CRISES:
AIDS & EVERYDAY

citizenship and identity form, while acknowledging political and material constraints. Articulation helps illuminate how sex worker organizations navigated political alliances with NGOs and activists in Bangalore and formed citizenship claims through those alliances.[6] So far, this book has focused on how NGOs, CBOs, and activist groups demanded and carved out a key role in HIV prevention programs that affected their lives. This chapter shifts the analytical focus to how these same organizations engaged in alliances outside of the AIDS realm, within their local political terrains. Focusing on sex worker organizations, this chapter shows that the AIDS response did not predetermine the kinds of citizenship assertions they could make. The hybrid spaces of the AIDS response meant that these groups were engaged not only in struggles over the practices of HIV prevention but also in a range of other local debates and demands around criminalization, stigma, and economic precarity.

ARTICULATING SEX WORKER POLITICS IN KOLKATA AND MAHARASHTRA

Sex worker organizations around India, as Chapter 3 showed, gained credibility and influence with local and national state officials by drawing on their alignments within the global AIDS field. But they also drew on local alliances with a wide array of social movements. In Kolkata, for example, DMSC's work required actively positioning itself within Kolkata's political milieu. When DMSC first formed, West Bengal was ruled by a Left Front government, led by the Communist Party (Marxist); in 2012, the Trinamool Congress (TMC) was voted into power.[7] While DMSC had more support within the Left Front government, as one interviewee put it, it "walked the rope" with both parties. He added, "We have not faced resistance, but some keep their distance. CPM doesn't accept sex work as labor. The party as a whole would never support us. We created spaces outside, through interactions and negotiations." This strategy of seeking out sources of support outside the party was relatively successful. Government officials gave a mixed response when their own beliefs about sex work were challenged. But DMSC worked to build the conditional spaces from which it could win the necessary party support. Outside observers agreed that DMSC managed to win support from political parties without identifying itself with any particular party. A member of DMSC was even invited to the swearing-in ceremony of

Mamata Banerjee, the leader of the TMC, as the new chief minister of West Bengal in 2011. The *Times of India* reported that Seema Fokla, the sex worker who had been invited, would be wearing a "green colour tant saree" and that Fokla and DMSC were "thankful to Didi [older sister] for showing a humane gesture by including sex workers in her invitee list."[8] DMSC had negotiated a tenuous point of inclusion into party politics.

DMSC also actively built social movement coalitions, particularly with women's and labor movements. As one feminist academic explained in an interview, while sex workers harbored some bitterness about the failure of a somewhat sexually conservative women's movement to address their concerns, by the mid-1990s a younger generation of feminists was more and more open to engaging sex workers. In 1992, an unprecedented meeting of sex workers with feminist activists took place at Jadavpur University, organized by the School of Women's Studies. "It was a powerful sight," she noted, "seeing those sex workers enter the academic space." At the same time, while DMSC interacted regularly with other women's movement activists in the city, one organizer noted that the connection was still loose: "We feel the women's movement is still an elite movement, with a weak connection to the grassroots." Relationships to the local labor movement were even more fragile, she said, but they evolved over time. While local trade union leaders were often uncomfortable with sex work, DMSC made inroads with the New Trade Union Initiative (NTUI), a coalition of nonparty-aligned trade unions, and by 2015, on my third visit, DMSC was leading NTUI's organizing efforts with women workers, including fisherwomen, domestic workers, and agricultural workers. Meanwhile, DMSC extended its presence in red-light districts, effectively challenging anti-trafficking organizations promoting an anti-sex-work stance.[9]

SANGRAM, in Sangli, Maharashtra, also took an approach to HIV prevention that evolved in relation to social movements. As one interviewee put it, "We are a set of NGOs who imagine we are movements, because some of us have come out of very structured movements . . . We bring in the principles of those movements into the NGOs." This movement orientation positioned SANGRAM to challenge coercive government measures and broaden participation. SANGRAM's approach to sex work evolved through a combination of local feminist ideologies, connections to global movements, and sex workers' own understandings of their work. In an interview, Meena Seshu, its general secretary, explained,

The reason SANGRAM is different is that it grew out of the feminist movement. So it's essentially the old feminist leftist principles that one believed in that helped build the ideology of SANGRAM. . . . the key strategies SANGRAM had written up long back, when we started this work, were self-determination, a woman-centered intervention. . . . when I say woman-centered I mean sex-worker–centered. Those days we didn't even have the word sex worker. We just said OK; women in sex work, women in prostitution, that was the language we used. . . . Terms were tough. We didn't want to use the commonly used negative connotations so we said OK let's place this in the fact that they're women. . . . the truth is that in India the construction of what is actually done is as a *dhandha* [business]. . . . But if you want to have some kind of links with the national, regional, global movements, if you don't have one terminology, the movement actually suffers. So with that in mind we just said OK, we accept sex work, because essentially we're saying that it is work.

As with DMSC, these alliances entailed an ongoing process of conflict and evolution. Seshu explained her relationships to feminist allies:

Since I came from the movement, and I had friends in the movement . . . my friends continued to be friends of mine. I mean they totally disapproved and disagreed with what I was doing. In fact, I was thrown out of a couple of meetings where I went and tried to speak about this. . . . I went underground with this issue for almost ten years. But I was continuing to talk with my friends. . . . my friends were . . . having these conversations with me, trying to understand what I had to say.

SANGRAM organized a series of conversations across the country, hosted by autonomous feminist organizations in major cities, including Bangalore, Delhi, Mumbai, and Pune, to engage in dialogue about sex work, opening up space for feminists to engage their discomfort and preconceptions. Seshu noted that this ongoing dialogue in informal spaces, through friendship and long-standing alliances, helped shape SANGRAM's principles as well as pushing mainstream feminists to take on sex workers' rights as a feminist issue. "We really worked at it," Seshu noted; alliances ensued from a process of struggle and negotiation.

SANGRAM's relationships with Dalit organizations were also complex. On the one hand, Dalit feminists who saw sex work as a form of gendered caste violence distrusted SANGRAM. Some members of Veshya Anyay Mukti Parishad (VAMP) came from *dēvadāsi* communities and were traditionally part of caste-based systems of prostitution. In their book *The Business of Sex*, Laxmi Murthy and Meena Seshu recount a presentation of a VAMP play written and performed by sex workers, some of whom were Dalit. After the play, several Dalit men challenged VAMP for presenting a false depiction of sex workers' lives and normalizing caste-based oppression. But Dalit sex workers within VAMP argued that they were "the Dalits among Dalits."[10] These negotiations reveal how sex worker organizations both shaped and were shaped by their alliances and conflicts with local social movements apart from the AIDS response.

ARTICULATING SEX WORKER, SEXUAL MINORITY, AND TRANSGENDER POLITICS IN BANGALORE

Bangalore provides a distinct geographic and political context for the articulation of social movements around gender and sexuality. Unlike in Kolkata, with its leftist political culture, in Bangalore the emergent sex worker movements had a more difficult time gaining traction with the language of workers' rights. Neither did they have centralized red-light areas in which sex workers lived and worked from brothels, nor hereditary forms of caste-based prostitution, such as the *dēvadāsi* system,[11] in which the foundations of kinship networks and informal community support systems might lay the groundwork for formal organizations. The pioneering organizing strategies of DMSC and SANGRAM could not be reproduced in Bangalore, where sex worker politics took shape in more heterogeneous ways.

Popular media characterizes Bangalore as a high-tech city, or India's Silicon Valley.[12] A recent report from Oxford Economics forecast Bangalore as the third-fastest-growing city in the world in 2019–2035.[13] Bangalore's economic growth has been dominated by the IT sector and the associated new global middle classes.[14] But Bangalore is also a regional hub for a growing number of migrant workers facing economic precarity and high costs of living.[15] In this context of fast, uneven growth and rising inequality, Bangalore receives large amounts of foreign funding for NGOs and associations: between 2002 and 2012, when I conducted my fieldwork, Bangalore usually received the second highest amount of foreign funding for associations among all cities in India (after Chennai), receiving about ₹812 crore, or US$135.2 million, in the 2011–2012 financial year.[16]

These economic and political conditions have particular implications for the articulation of feminist and queer politics in the city. A BJP-dominated city, Bangalore has what several interviewees considered a technocratic, NGO-ized social sector, with a small left largely disconnected from electoral politics.[17] Though Bangalore has had a history of trade unionism and garment worker strikes led by women, the spatial organization of the city and its tradition of public sector employment have meant a middle-class culture and the growing invisibilization of working-class people.[18] The women's movement in Bangalore has been smaller than in India's larger cities but has been defined by the same kind of "NGO crowding" that shapes Karnataka's social sector overall.[19] Bangalore hosts queer NGOs that are nationally prominent and is the destination for queer and transgender migrants from the neighboring states of Tamil Nadu, Kerala, and Andhra Pradesh, as well as from rural and small-town Karnataka.[20] While often referred to as Pub City, Bangalore's growing middle classes, call centers, and English-speaking elite have emerged alongside a backlash to globalization, tied both to linguistic and regional nationalism. Bangalore has been the site of draconian moral policing tied to this backlash, such as a ban on dancing in bars. The city is the site of deep tensions about gender, sexuality, and globalization.[21] In the context of the AIDS crisis, then, Bangalore provided the conditions for a range of divergent political articulations, from leftist queer orientations to consultancies run by former techies to everything in between.

The history of formal organization among sex workers and sexual minority groups in Bangalore is entangled both with these particular dynamics of economic and social transformation and the dynamics of the AIDS response. In 1993, the NGO Samraksha, an offshoot of the NGO Samuha, began working in the area of AIDS in Karnataka. Samraksha played a role in sex worker, sexual minority, and transgender organizing in Bangalore. In the early phases, Samraksha's director began as a volunteer in government STI clinics, supporting people informally when they tested positive for HIV. As she explored possibilities for broadening Samraksha's work, she went to visit the South India AIDS Action Programme in Chennai, founded two years earlier, and, building from there, began work with sex workers in Bangalore.

Another organization, Sadhana Mahila Gumpu, formed around 2001, led by a former peer educator at Samraksha. Largely autonomous, Sadhana drew financial and institutional support from feminist organizers and the Alternative Law Forum, a collective of progressive lawyers. These groups formed the starting point for later sex worker organizing in the city.

Compared to sex worker organizing, the formation of sexual minority and transgender organizations in Bangalore was more indirectly linked to the AIDS response, but the two areas of activism developed in tandem. In 1994, Good as You, a group of predominantly middle-class, English-speaking gay men, formed, first meeting at a member's home and later in the Samraksha office. (The same year, Humsafar Trust[22] and the Naz Foundation,[23] two other organizations working with gay men and conducting AIDS programs, formed in Mumbai and Delhi, respectively.) In 1999, two new sexual minority organizations formed in Bangalore: Sangama[24] and Swabhava.[25] Sangama initially focused on documenting human rights abuses against sexual minorities and had more of a middle-class, English-speaking constituency.[26] Over time, a group of working-class kothis and *hijras*[27] began to meet at Sangama's office, under the name Snehashraya. In 2000, the police began an effort to seek out kothis in the city and started detaining them, and Snehashraya members stopped coming to Sangama, fearing arrest. Sangama formally registered in 2001 and began a Sunday drop-in center for working-class sexual minorities in 2002.[28]

During the next several years, Sangama leaders decided to focus on working-class sexual minorities in Bangalore. Legal aid and advocacy against police violence became a major focus, and in 2002, Sangama submitted a memorandum to the chief minister against police violence against sex workers. These shifts caused some rifts among Sangama's members. As part of a coalition called the Forum for Sex Workers' Rights, they also held a public protest at Town Hall. Police violence became a key point of commonality across transgender women, cisgender women, and kothi sex workers. But the group that met on Sundays also began to participate in other local activism, through the Narmada Solidarity Forum and the People's Initiative for Peace, for example, and formed an autonomous organization called Vividha.[29] In 2003, the Peoples' Union for Civil Liberties, Karnataka, in collaboration with the Alternative Law Forum, Sangama, Vimochana, and other local activist groups published a path-breaking collaborative report documenting human rights violations against kothi and hijra sex workers in Bangalore, including against people involved in HIV prevention. The report made a strong challenge to the legal and political marginalization of kothi and hijra sex workers, as well as documenting the vibrant space of sexual minority activism in Bangalore at the time.[30] Sangama also helped set up a shelter for female-born sexual minorities. In the years after, several further groups formed. LesBiT, a group of female-born sexual minorities, formed in 2005 after breaking away from Sangama and offered several important critiques of NGO-driven activism;[31] Payana, another group focused on working-class LGBTQIA+ issues, formed in 2009.[32] The space of sexual minority activism in Bangalore, in short, was a rich space of debate, as well as alliances with other social movements.

When the Gates Foundation's Avahan program arrived in 2003, in a partnership with the state government that promised to massively scale up HIV prevention programs for sex workers and sexual minority groups in Bangalore and across South India, both groups had already been in the process of organizing for more than a decade, Samraksha for HIV prevention and Sangama for sex worker, sexual minority, and transgender activism. Avahan infused money, monitoring and evaluation requirements, and new institutional access into this emerging organizational context, raising the stakes and introducing new debates and conflicts.

NAVIGATING THE STATE AND DONORS IN THE ERA OF LARGE-SCALE AIDS PROGRAMS

When the Gates Foundation began its work in India, it had little experience engaging with community organizations. The director of the Gates Foundation's India program, Ashok Alexander, came to HIV prevention from a long career at McKinsey. In his 2018 book, *A Stranger Truth,* he describes his early efforts to learn about HIV in India as "plunging into the vast unknown, with no parachute, no map."[33] Given this unfamiliarity, the Gates Foundation necessarily built on existing organizational landscapes of HIV prevention and sex worker, sexual minority, and transgender organizing. Nationally, DMSC, which "proved to the world that programs can successfully engage most-at-risk populations (MARPS)," formed an "important inspiration" for Gates planners.[34] Locally, the Gates Foundation and state agencies drew on NGOs, CBOs, and activists with experience and with access to high-risk groups.

Because Karnataka was considered to have a high HIV prevalence—1.7% of pregnant women in the state tested positive for HIV in 2002, and one researcher told me in an interview they believed Karnataka to be "the next epicenter of the epidemic"[35]—the Gates Foundation included Karnataka as one of its focus states.[36] In Bangalore, targeted interventions were organized into seven geographic zones, with a combination of a CBO and an NGO conducting HIV prevention outreach in each zone. Targeted interventions for each of the three high-risk groups—female sex workers, men who have sex with men, and IV drug users—were run separately, by separate organizations. By the mid-2000s, several new organizations of sex workers, sexual minorities, and transgender people took shape, including Swathi Mahila Sangha, Vijaya Mahila Sangha, Jyothi Mahila Sangha, and Samara. Several leaders of these organizations came from organizations that had worked in HIV prevention starting in the 1990s, but now they were part of the new statewide infrastructure.

Organizations in Bangalore pursued a wide range of programs. In addition to the work of HIV prevention, which included regular outreach, condom distribution, and running drop-in centers with clinics, CBOs formed cooperative societies, began catering and tailoring businesses, responded to crisis calls when a sex worker was arrested or detained by police, and participated in advocacy. For example, the largest of these CBOs, Swathi Mahila Sangha, operates a microenterprise program that provides financial services to eleven thousand sex workers, and its partner, Swasti Health Catalyst, works nationally and globally.[37] Outside of these more formal efforts, I also observed a range of informal support systems—intervening in family disputes; talking to family members about sexuality; helping organize a daughter's wedding; or holding birthday parties, baby showers, and naming ceremonies. Empowerment and addressing violence became core aims, while HIV prevention work appeared as simply an everyday obligation, a basic responsibility required to keep the organization running. One CBO leader explained, "At home, first we send the children to school, get them ready, and then send the husband [to work], and then we eat a little and do the housework. It's like that. If I look at this priority [on HIV prevention programs], I think of it like that." For her, fulfilling the mandated tasks of AIDS programs recalled the patriarchal obligations of middle-class domestic life. AIDS programs, the "husband and children," represented the basic tasks one must complete as a housewife; after sending them off, she could focus on getting her own house in order, "eating a little" and conducting programs for women's empowerment. She did not see it as her role to challenge the structure of this metaphorical household. But she saw community work as a necessary step to doing HIV prevention work effectively. As an activist put it: "HIV is not the only issue in the community. There's more beyond HIV. There's a lot more needs to be done to accept yourself. . . . Self-respect. Self-dignity. If you have these, you automatically use a condom. Automatically you can prevent HIV/AIDS!"

Alongside these approaches to HIV prevention programs that sought to broaden the terms on which HIV prevention was conceptualized and delivered, others were more openly critical of sex workers, sexual minorities, and transgender people being labeled vectors of disease.[38] At the same time, as one NGO leader recalled, "people were dying," and the funding offered an opportunity to reach constituents at a large scale, to "get in and change the game." As HIV prevention initiatives increasingly began to overwhelm other activist work, debates and conflicts continued. One activist told me, "We were very very wary of HIV funding. . . . and it is because we have been constantly on guard that we were able to survive. And now the Gates Foundation is going away . . . . So much money can really destroy things, but somehow we were able to prevent it."

One organization, the Karnataka Sex Workers' Union, formed explicitly to present an oppositional voice, in collaboration with Sangama and other labor and leftist movement groups. The Union formed in response to the arrests of four sex workers in Channapatna, a town outside Bangalore, in 2006. When the women were detained for three months, the newly formed Union, a mix of employees of Sangama and another HIV prevention NGO called Suraksha, held protests outside the local police station until they were released. The Union formally announced its presence with a rally on May Day. The Union also protested a local TV station for releasing the names and images of sex workers without their consent.[39] "[HIV prevention] doesn't come into our work," one Union leader said in an interview. "What we care about is that we want our [sex] work to be recognized as work."

The Union openly protested AIDS programs. For example, in 2010, it organized a surprise protest at the government-sponsored World AIDS Day event, standing up in the audience with red umbrellas, symbolic of the international sex workers' movement, in objection to breaches of confidentiality, the director of the state AIDS prevention society's "rude and insulting behavior," and coercive testing practices. The Union held rallies to protest part-time work appointments for HIV peer educators, arguing that they violated labor rights.

On the other hand, the Union used creative strategies to work within AIDS programs. The Union formed as an independent organization with its own elected board, and, in 2008, applied for trade union registration. (The same year, Sangama joined other organizations in the Coalition for Sex Workers and Sexuality Minority Rights to organize Bangalore's first Pride Parade.) Staff from Sangama registered themselves independently as paying members of the Union. A mandated event for sensitization of police or pimps would be followed by a Union protest or rally. Members would mark the difference between the organizations, and the Union's independence from AIDS programs, by taking down the AIDS program banner and putting up a new one announcing the event was now a Union event. Union staff visited HIV prevention offices to recruit members and update them on new developments. The Union thus built strategically on AIDS organizational infrastructure even as it challenged its premise.

The Union's position as simultaneously part of and outside of the AIDS infrastructure gave it a unique strategic vantage point from which to challenge abuses within NGOs. One afternoon I visited a sex worker who worked for a local NGO. She sat tying flowers into a string while she complained to me about her job as an HIV peer educator. "They talk to you badly," she said. "I told them, you exist because of us, so what's the point if you treat us badly? You're getting your livelihood out of us. I told them exactly that." She had a clear sense of her importance to the NGO. A year later, the Union protested the NGO, threatened to call in the media, and wrote letters to the state agency for AIDS prevention. Rapidly, funds to the NGO were withdrawn and management turned over to a different organization. The Union's activist orientation, and links to activists in the city, combined with state AIDS officials' dependence on sex worker organizations to create an unusual responsiveness to sex workers' complaints.

TO CLAP OR NOT TO CLAP

One key point of variation among sex worker, sexual minority, and transgender organizations, then, hinged on how they related to HIV prevention programs—collaboratively or oppositionally, or somewhere in between. But organizations and individual activists also varied in their long-term aims. For some organizations, the main task was to improve the economic standing of sex workers through a combination of state and private mechanisms. For others, the condition for any such improvement was the recognition of sex work as work. These differences were articulated through organizations' distinct relationships with the organizational landscape of Bangalore's social movements.

At least two organizations working with cisgender women sex workers in Bangalore aimed to develop independent social enterprises that would allow them, as they put it, to stand on their own feet. This pursuit of independence applied to both individual entrepreneurship—supported through microfinance programs—and organizational autonomy through microenterprises that could help fund organizational activities. Within this framework, as one interviewee put it, the state's "grand programs" were not reliable sources of support. These organizations also worked to improve access to existing social entitlements by, for example, helping sex workers apply for voter identification cards and ration cards. These efforts helped sex workers access the state's existing protection systems for poor women.

For more activist organizations, the state was the target of protest, either as a perpetrator of violence or as a provider of social welfare. Union activists regularly responded to instances of police violence or the illegal detainment of sexual minorities or sex workers, not just by supporting individual sex workers who had been detained but also by holding public protests and turning to the media.[40] They used protest tactics to demand social welfare from the state—universal old-age pensions; fair pay for HIV prevention workers; subsidized housing for HIV-positive people, sex workers, and transgender people; government employment—and they did so explicitly as sex workers organizing as workers.

These divergent approaches to making demands on the state reflected divergent articulations of sex worker identity. At several sex worker CBOs I visited, members rarely referred to themselves as sex worker's organizations but simply as women's groups. When I asked one sex worker leader why sex work was not included in her organization's name, she explained that, because sex work was intertwined with other aspects of women's lives, emphasizing sex work alone was reductive. She distinguished her organization's approach to women's lives from an approach that centered the rights of sex

DEMANDING THINGS FROM THE STATE

workers. Once, I asked her what she thought of sex worker activists in Kolkata, who organized out of red-light districts and demanded recognition from the state as workers. She was critical: "We come in the morning, we work, we eat with our children and we go to sleep with peace of mind, wake up, and come again. There [in Kolkata] it's not like that. . . . They don't even know how to cook, the people who stay there. They don't know what a family is. Client, sex, condom, other than that, what do they know in red-light areas? They don't know how to dress neatly. At festival time they can't celebrate properly." Her aversion to sex worker activism in Kolkata indicated her discomfort not only with activist demands but also activist lifestyles. A sex worker activist in Kolkata, she suggested, did not eat with her children, cook, understand family, dress well, or celebrate festivals. A sex worker activist was a sex worker but not a respectable woman. Her location in a red-light district cut her off from the peace and stability of the household and rendered her visibly transgressive. Her aversion to public transgression extended to transgender women in sex work. "For us it's about being a mother and taking care of our children. For them it's going everywhere and clapping," she once said to me of transgender activists as we ate lunch. A key aspect of a hijra's cultural repertoire is to clap her hands while begging for change at street intersections, so clapping encapsulated both transgressive sexuality and transgressive demands for resources.

Some NGO workers opposed activists who, as one interviewee put it, "think sex work is a right." "NNSW thinks sex work is a right. They should be given workers' rights. It's labor. Fine, but many of the sex workers . . . back home are not known as sex workers . . . they are wives, they are daughters, they are daughters-in-law, they are sisters to somebody. For neighbors they are nurses, for neighbors they are domestic maids. Now why would I tag and say look, I'm a sex worker, give me labor rights?" This account emphasized sex workers' family lives, and emphasized eschewing visibility. He avoided what he called "shouting and screaming," or, as another interviewee put it, "going on TV" and "yelling on the roof that we are sex workers." Of course, these impressions did not square with the reality of Kolkata sex worker activists who do have children and celebrate festivals or who do not live in red-light areas at all. But they do clarify the contrast some sex worker organizations placed between transgressive activism and self-reliance, gendered respectability, and what they called soft advocacy over public protest.

Sadhana, an autonomous organization, was distinct from these collectives in that it did not become involved in the AIDS response at all. Sadhana initially drew financial and administrative support from organizers then working at Vimochana, a feminist organization; the Alternative Law Forum and the People's Union for Civil Liberties-Karnataka (PUCL-K); and later from Jana Sahayog, CIEDS, and Gamana Mahila Samuha. Sadhana charted a path that both rejected the biomedical approach and quantitative documentation demands of HIV prevention programs and avoided assuming that the term *sex work* was always meaningful to women, as one interviewee explained. Early on, Sadhana referred to its members as women in sex work and prostitution, rather than sex workers, and used the term *gumpu* [group] rather than *sangha* [association.][41] This approach was deliberately cautious about imposing categorizations that did not speak to women who did not identify with the term *sex worker*, as well as members' experience of diverse occupations that could not be defined by sex work alone. "A sex worker on the street does sex, and so does a housewife at home," one leader explained to me. As Sadhana grew as an organization and engaged with sex worker activists nationally, and its members came to identify with the terminology, Sadhana began to use the term *sex work* in its advocacy.

Sadhana members met weekly during the time of my fieldwork. While NGO allies paid the staff and donated space, they did not regularly attend meetings or lead activities. At the time, everyday activities at Sadhana extended from the relations of work on the street, resolving conflicts among women, discussing problems with clients, and supporting women who had been detained by police. Members also accompanied other sex workers to the hospital if they needed support and had helped trafficked children get out of the industry. In collaboration with the Alternative Law Forum, between 2001 and 2006 they fought 575 cases of women who were arrested and falsely accused by the police, and they won 375 of them, resulting in the Karnataka Police issuing a reminder to all police stations not to arrest sex workers under the ITPA.[42] Sadhana members attended events protesting the abuse of Dalit sweepers; participated in a forum against forced evictions in the city; and, along with sexual minority groups, the Union, Dalit groups, and other leftist groups in the city, signed on to a letter condemning the moral policing of sex workers.[43] Sadhana works independently from NGOs, except for administrative support from the NGO Jana Sahayog. It continues to address violence on the street and at home, support sex workers' children, assist sex workers navigating the healthcare system, and help women and children who have been trafficked. It even staged a dramatic performance about sex workers' lives. It has become a leading activist voice for sex workers in the state, advocating for state schemes to support sex workers and women and allying with activists and social justice NGOs.

The Union, in contrast to these other organizations, made the concept of sex work as work central to its advocacy from the outset. One staff member of the Union explained the difference between the Union and women's groups who worked with sex workers: "For auto [rickshaw] drivers, there's a union, for lorry [truck] drivers, there's a union. Various people have made unions. We're sex workers. We also made a union." While other sex worker organizers interpreted the dispersed nature of sex work in Bangalore as a reason to downplay sex worker identity, Union members saw it as a justification to highlight it. A board member explained,

> I thought I was the only one, but when I saw those women, I saw that there are so many people. My community is facing so much difficulty. Let's join with them, let's clap with them loudly, let the sound be heard, let the government hear our sound. No one can hear the sound of one person, but if we all clap, people gather, wondering what's happening. . . . We don't need any other name than sex worker. That's what we're doing. [She compares the phrase *sex worker* to the names of Dalit groups that have been reclaimed.] We're sex workers. Yes, we do sex work. What's wrong with that?

For some, then, clapping was threatening, reminiscent of the hijra practice of clapping when panhandling at traffic intersections, and at odds with being a good mother. For others, clapping became the basis for solidarity to make demands on the state from a shared platform.[44]

The Union defined sex workers in way that included sexual minorities and transgender people, though cisgender women still made up the bulk of its membership.[45] One kothi member explained, "And some of the problems were almost one, and in some areas there were differences . . . Female sex workers had children. Our people [e.g., kothis] don't have children . . . but in sex work, violence, or [those kinds of] problems, when all that came up, it was mostly similar. When we discussed it, we said the work we are doing is respectable work and we wanted it recognized as work . . . So then we said OK, and we started the Union." Most of my interviewees who were Union members, including cisgender women members, saw this alliance as beneficial. The Union supported national organizing for sexual minority rights and activism against Section 377 of the Indian Penal Code,[46] but it also intervened in more immediate situations of police brutality against sexual minorities in Bangalore.

The identity card the Union provided its members was a particular assertion of citizenship that centered sex worker identity. A Union board member recalled its effects:

> They gave me an identity card. I took it and went around for two days. And now no one would come near me. Everyone said you've become a big person now madam; you won't talk to all of us now. . . . Wherever I went. [Since then] I haven't faced injustice, nothing has happened anywhere. I do the work [sex work]. I do it practically twenty-four hours a day. But I haven't had anything happen to me at all. [Why?] Because before I was afraid. Of who would come, who would scare me, hit me, shout at me. Of who would see me. . . . When I got the license, it felt like hey, I'm doing the work, look, let me show you my card. I got courage when the sex worker union came. Now I have courage. Now I can stand up to all of them.

The identity card physically manifested her identity as a sex worker, linking her to other sex workers as a basis for asserting everyday rights.[47] It became a practical tool for citizenship.

The divergent positions among Bangalore sex worker organizations on how to make demands on the state evolved in relation to local political struggles. A Union ally noted, "I definitely come from a left-leaning background. So, it was very interesting for us to put class right up in front. Poverty, working-class issues, social exclusion. . . . we can build that solidarity with other people which is what we think is critical for any social change." In practice, the Union's alliances were sometimes precarious. For example, several interviewees explained that some domestic worker organizers were wary of the stigma of association with sex workers. I once attended an anti-trafficking training with two Union activists during which several participants challenged the possibility that anyone could willingly participate in sex work. The activists, nevertheless, calmly stood up and introduced themselves as sex workers in Kannada, though the entire meeting had been conducted in English. In an interview, a Dalit feminist ally described her reservations about sex work as a form of stigmatized work in which Dalit women were disproportionately engaged, even as she said she agreed with sex workers' right to do sex work. The Union worked to sustain their relationships. "They are regular attenders of meetings," an ally from a garment workers' union noted. Today, a Union representative is the vice president of the National Network of Sex Workers (NNSW).

These distinct orientations to sex work were articulated in relation to local struggles. While a history of alliances with leftist groups helped inform the Union's coalition politics, Sadhana Mahila Gumpu developed a distinct position on sex work through feminist alliances and the dynamics of sex work on the street. Other collectives in Bangalore built on their relationships to HIV prevention programs and entrepreneurial NGO initiatives for women's empowerment and were less involved in activism or in centering sex worker identity.

GENDER, SEXUALITY, AND CITIZENSHIP

With good reason, scholars have pointed to the ways in which AIDS programs homogenize and depoliticize sexual marginalization.[48] These scholars suggest that the AIDS industry limits the possibilities for those at the heart of AIDS programs to form political demands.[49] AIDS programs helped set the institutional and financial context for organizing on the basis of sexuality in Bangalore starting in the early 1990s, first through smaller-scale NGO efforts, later through government programs, and eventually within the Gates Foundation's Avahan initiative. While some organizations strove to remain outside the ambit of AIDS programs, or even protest them, and others were central to their functioning, it was difficult for any organization working with sex workers, sexual minorities, and transgender people in Bangalore during this period to ignore AIDS and the institutional infrastructure it brought with it.

Nevertheless, this chapter has shown that these organizations of sex workers, sexual minorities, and transgender people were also engaged in numerous other local struggles, and through those struggles, articulated diverse claims on the state. Organizations of sex workers, sexual minorities, and transgender people involved in the AIDS response built on local activist infrastructures that were entangled with HIV prevention but could not be reduced to it. As AIDS programs scaled up and organizations evolved, they developed a widely varied set of practices within this heterogeneous milieu.

Some organizations sought state recognition by positioning themselves as just as respectable as other (non-sex-working, cisgender) women—while cultivating the entrepreneurial skills to stand on their own feet. Their challenge to the AIDS establishment lay precisely in their identification with gendered respectability: members insisted they were not primarily carriers of disease but rather savvy mothers and daughters who could run a massive, efficient public health program. In a more oppositional relationship to AIDS programs, Union members made claims on the state as workers. They aligned themselves with other groups oppressed by class and caste domination and state violence—sexual minorities, Dalits, informal workers, and their intersections.

The diversity of articulations of sex worker politics in the shadow of AIDS was not limited to the organizational terrain of Bangalore. It also played out nationally. Reflecting on one national meeting of sex worker activists working within the AIDS response, one interviewee noted, "The schism in the sex work movement became apparent. There was [DMSC] and others, who all believe in the trade union and activism approach. . . . Then there is a set of NGOs and iNGOs [international NGOs], including KHPT . . . [that] believe that there is a role for . . . program advocacy." A joint proposal to the Global Fund, written by NGOs from across India, bears the clear marks of this debate. While parts of the proposal critique "coercive NGO practices" and the tendency of health interventions to "stigmatize women in sex work by labeling them as the source of infection,"[50] other parts of the proposal argue that "some of the CBOs get into an activist mode and do not feel the need for addressing risk reduction as need for the community, but focus only on rights to the exclusion of all other issues."[51]

Despite the differences, however, these varied organizations, in their own ways, moved beyond the logic of containment that defined India's early AIDS response, as well as beyond the logic of incorporation that saw them as integral of the AIDS response but invisible outside of it. Even as they diverged over advocacy or protest, transgressive or respectable sexuality, or even the metaphorical virtues of clapping as political practice, they expanded the range of questions AIDS programs must engage. By extending the analytical focus beyond the scope within which AIDS programs were initially defined to include the range of local political alliances different organizations pursued, this chapter has shown how the state AIDS management practices around deviant sexuality could be differentially rearticulated.

While the various organizations involved in the AIDS response charted distinct political trajectories, in the lives of sex workers, sexual minorities, and transgender people, they often overlapped. "I know all the offices," one peer educator at a sex worker CBO told me, as I listed various organizations in the city. Most members of the Union also worked for other CBOs as peer educators or outreach workers. Together, these organizational engagements occasioned not only group claims and collective solidarities but also more personal transformations. As they worked in HIV prevention programs, sex workers, sexual minorities, and transgender people learned new ways of embodying sexuality, and new ways of relating to each other as well as to the state. The next chapter turns to these transformations, examining how the AIDS crisis opened up new opportunities for self-making for those who inhabited it.

5 | RISKY SELVES

EARLY IN PREETHI'S career as a sex worker, she was often dragged to the police station and beaten by police. At one point, she said, they wouldn't let her stand anywhere in the Majestic bus stand, where she went every evening for sex work. But as time passed, these violent encounters became less frequent. Preethi said it was because she had changed. Sitting on the breezy terrace of the NGO office where she worked as an HIV prevention outreach worker, just as the afternoon light began to fade, she explained, "Now I kind of hold a bag, and I don't wear as much makeup. Before, I'd wear a deep-necked dress, thinking I needed it for sex work. Now the way I think about it is, if they [clients] come, let them come, but if not, no. If he wants it, he'll take me no matter what. But before, I used to fall all over their bodies, asking, 'will you come with me?'" Preethi was describing a change in her everyday embodiment as a sex worker. Once sexually demonstrative as she sought clients at Majestic, Preethi had developed a more aloof, self-contained, middle-class feminine persona. She'd now stand holding a handbag—her ticket to a purposeful, respectable presence in public space—blending into the background, and waiting for clients to come to her. She avoided appearing to be there for sex; she now made sure to look like she had other things to do. I asked Preethi why she had changed in this way. She explained:

I feel it's not as important. We need money for our difficulties, but we shouldn't exist for money. I've learned a little. Before I used to spend a lot on clothing. I'd buy the cloth in the morning, get it stitched in the afternoon, and wear that outfit and go out that evening. The neck would be this deep, and I'd pull the veil up like this [she showed me how she had once arranged her *dupatta* (scarf) to show off her breasts.] Back then, that was my only job. Sex work was my only way of earning. . . . But now, I don't make the neck deep. I go and sit at the bar. I start drinking. And they [clients] come to me on their own . . . . I say I work in an HIV prevention NGO. And if they're interested, they say come with me, madam, and I have a lodge I usually go to, so I take them there.

That Preethi mentioned HIV prevention work when soliciting clients for sex work might seem unusual, but not if we consider the importance it held in Preethi's self-formation. Preethi was no longer "only" a sex worker: she now worked at an office. Working in an HIV prevention job that was premised on her membership in a high-risk group of transgender sex workers had, unexpectedly, offered her a route to loosening her reliance on sex work:

After we [transgender women] have come outside, we're coming to realize we also have the capacity to work. . . . We didn't used to come outside at all. Watch TV, cook, eat. Is it five o'clock in the evening? Take a bath, and come to Majestic. That's all we knew. I thought the whole universe was just this. When I came to an NGO, I gained a little discipline [*shistu*]. Because I go around on the bus, I have to be a bit decent . . . I sit in the front seats [those reserved for women], and if anyone near me asks me for directions, I kind of talk in a slow, soft voice. "This way, aunty." [Preethi talks in a soft voice, eyes downcast, as she evokes her conversation with her seatmate.]. . . . Before, I wouldn't wake up until one in the afternoon. Since coming to the office, [I've learned] timings. If I have to be at the office at twelve thirty, I get up at ten and get ready. If they tell us we have to come at ten for a meeting, the night before I set an alarm and remember that I have to get up at eight itself. So that's changed.

It was the first of several conversations Preethi and I would have over the next five years, sitting in the NGO office, walking around her neighborhood, or in her apartment, where I sat curled up on a bench and she poured dosa after dosa for me to eat. Preethi was a transgender woman who had once been part of the hijra community. When she found a partner who promised to support her financially, she left the community. When the partner broke his promise, she fell into a deep depression. It was then that she found herself working in HIV prevention: she asked for a job at the drop-in center where she had been spending time, explaining to the program manager there that getting out of the house was her only way to escape her loneliness.

For Preethi, the AIDS crisis that splashed across Indian headlines in the 1990s was a distant aspect of her everyday life. Instead, AIDS mattered because of the organizational spaces it had created. The NGO had allowed Preethi to "come outside."[1] It had given Preethi new sources of income, a newly expansive sense of her access to public space, and a new way of organizing her time. She had gained confidence talking to police officers about sex work: "After I joined the office," she said, "I got a little more courage and talked to the police. What's wrong with working?" Simultaneous with these transformations was one more intangible: she had learned to inhabit gendered respectability, to cover her breasts, speak softly, and look like she had something else to do. She had learned to leverage this respectability at the right times and play with its boundaries at other times—alone, she was carefully demure; when she was with friends, she was louder, joking with them at the back of the bus. The organization of her time had changed too. As a peer educator, she had cut down on sex work. Sex work was no longer her "only way of earning." Her office work appeased her family, who worried that as a sex worker she would "get some disease." All this amounted to a new way of moving through the world, a new embodiment and practice of gender, class, and sexuality. When she'd lived in the hijra community, she told me, "I used to be rough . . . because they [the others in her house] were all Tamilians. They were all loud." Now, she told me, she had changed in ways people would describe to me over and over as I conducted my fieldwork: "I used to be rough before, but now I've become smooth."[2]

In this chapter, I trace what Preethi meant when she—and many of my other interviewees, including cisgender men and women and transgender women—described "becoming smooth." I argue that, as sex workers, men who have sex with men, kothis, hijras, and transgender women became incorporated into the AIDS response, and into the new political articulations that ensued, and they learned new ways of naming, embodying, and practicing sexuality. NGO practices encouraged HIV prevention workers, on the one hand, to be respectable in ways that circumscribed transgressive sexuality (as in Preethi's lighter makeup and her handbag), and on the other, to speak openly about sexuality in the right contexts and at the right times (as in her willingness to challenge police authority). AIDS programs reinforced these ideals through naming practices shaped by epidemiological classification, diversified income, and the experience of the HIV prevention drop-in center, or "office," where emerging sexual subjectivities were practiced in a safe and intimate space. But people like Preethi also subverted this ideal. While organizations varied widely in the kinds of collective claims they articulated, as Chapter 4 showed, they all offered avenues to personal transformation. Drop-in centers became hybrid sites of state surveillance, collective articulation, and personal care and self-making.

Preethi's account complicates existing accounts of the AIDS industry, both critical and celebratory. Scholars have long noted the dangers of AIDS cosmopolitanism, or the imposition of oversimplified global sexual categories on more complex realities of sexual practice.[3] These arguments assume that the state and donors exist in a realm somehow distinct from everyday life, that there is some authentic truth beyond them. But as Lawrence Cohen argues in his genealogy of the kothi category, even indigenous categories are produced through transnational processes and battles over authenticity.[4] Meanwhile, government officials I interviewed often suggested AIDS programs were a liberating force in the lives of high-risk groups and that it was because of AIDS programs that these groups had been empowered."[5]

In contrast to accounts of AIDS programs as colonizing or liberating sexuality, scholars like Celeste Watkins-Hayes have written about how AIDS programs—and AIDS activism—can become the basis for "remaking a life," for building new structures of resilience and connection.[6] This chapter focuses on how AIDS changed the landscape for embodying and practicing sexuality for high-risk groups through everyday life. Like the pious women in Saba Mahmood's account of Islamic practice in Egypt, the HIV prevention workers in this study engaged in a process of disciplined self-formation.[7] They used the body as a developable means toward the formation of an ideal HIV prevention target, one who was both respectable enough to blend in and confident enough to make demands. This chapter grapples with ways in which sex workers, sexual minorities, and transgender people learn, inhabit, and subvert gendered and sexual norms within the hybrid spaces of HIV prevention.

Preethi admired smoothness in those she met. Once, as we were leaving her flat, she said, "I like how you are—so soft, so silent and smooth." She, too, was usually smooth, she said, but when she spent time with her hijra friends, she became more rough. "If I'm with you, I can learn things from you. I think, look, Gowri's so silent; I can be like that. I change if I'm with the [hijra] community." Preethi was pointing to the pedagogy of sexual embodiment and feminine respectability that she had sought out for herself, that she saw in me, a middle-class, English-speaking, dominant-caste cisgender woman. Preethi admired transgender women activists who spoke fluent English and could interact with foreign visitors at her NGO. As an HIV prevention worker, Preethi sought to manage her sexuality in ways that allowed her to make political demands as transgender while not endangering her claim to gendered respectability. Indeed, she had learned to cultivate this style of sexual embodiment, like the smoothness I represented to her. Yet this process was always uneven and contradictory; smoothness was not always the only goal, and it was often a topic of debate or tension. Preethi had transformed herself, but she had also learned when and how smoothness could be troubled or suspended.

Smoothness was not simply superficial vocabulary imposed by biomedical science on a deeper, more radical, or more authentic sexual truth. Becoming a subject of HIV prevention initiatives offered a new grammar of bodily practice,[8] a new field of possibilities that allowed Preethi to cultivate, unevenly, a smoother life.[9] It was not worn lightly; it was stitched into the cut of her neckline, the pitch of her voice, the cast of her eyes, and the rhythm of her morning. Through HIV prevention work, Preethi came to embody a new kind of self.[10]

THE IDEAL HIV PREVENTION TARGET

The persona of the ideal HIV prevention target my interviewees cultivated rarely meant they *stopped* doing sex work or having sex with men—the risk behaviors that defined them as eligible for HIV prevention programs. Rather, it meant *how* they did these things changed: HIV prevention programs idealized subtler shifts in sexual practices. These ideals became clear in my interview with Aparna, a member of a community-based organization that did HIV prevention with women in sex work. Aparna had been introduced to sex work by her mother-in-law. Her mother-in-law had initially been nervous about asking Aparna to do sex work because, she said, she was from a "good family," and Aparna herself had been reluctant. But as her husband's drinking problems got worse and she began to struggle to support her children, Aparna had changed her mind. Nevertheless, she was careful to keep her work private. No one on her side of the family knew what she did. "I don't actually come outside at all," she said; she communicated with clients over the phone and did sex work indoors. If she had to go somewhere to meet a client, she didn't even take the bus; she preferred to pay more for a private auto-rickshaw. When I asked what she thought her CBO should focus on, she said:

> They should be able to help women. There are so many women like us. Now, I do [sex work] fearfully, but some are without fear; they go to the [City] Market, wearing makeup, wearing those blouses like this, and wearing saris like this [she indicates clothing that shows off the body.] When I see all that I feel disgusted [*asahya*]. . . . Do it [sex work]; there's nothing wrong in it. But do it neatly. . . . What's inside should be inside; it shouldn't come outside. . . . Do it at home as much as you can. Why do you have to be in the street?

The space of the office allowed sex work to be done "inside" in the way Aparna described: one could sit in the office, take calls, and coordinate clients instead of soliciting in public. But Aparna's entreaty was also a moral one. She suggested that sex workers could do sex work, that women often must do it to survive, but that it should be done "neatly." As Aditi, another long-time member of the same CBO, put it, "You should do it secretly, without people knowing. It should be something people don't know, that you do for your survival. This is the wisdom they gave us [at the CBO]."[11] Sex work was not itself morally wrong, but it should be done discreetly, and it should not affect a woman's respectable public persona; it should not mean wearing makeup or a low-cut blouse.

Aparna's preference for doing sex work "neatly" was reflected in the sartorial practices I noticed in some sex worker CBOs. Those higher up in the CBO hierarchy wore fashionable silk saris with gold jewelry and flowers in their hair. "It's fine to wear old clothes, but they shouldn't be dirty," a staff member, Shakuntala, once whispered to me about an errant peer educator at the office. Once, as I stood in a meeting, several women called me over into the corner, whispering to me that there was a small tear in my top and I should immediately go home and change. I was often given advice about how to wear my *dupatta* or encouraged to wear a sari. I eventually learned that these practices helped maintain a carefully observed boundary between respectable and unrespectable women, between women who were known to be sex workers and women who blended in. In some cases, this negotiation was a strategic one that protected the office from criticism, or even being shut down. Once, as I sat at a CBO office on the outskirts of the city, one of the CBO leaders called a member to ask her to come to the office. "Not her, please," said Kashi, one of the outreach workers. "She's always drunk. Please don't bring her or we'll get kicked out of the office." "Isn't this office for the community?" I asked, curious. Kashi was apologetic. "The landlords know her and she drinks in public. She does sex work everywhere and everyone knows. She's become noted." In this office that existed to serve the health needs of sex workers, the fact that someone was known to be a sex worker made her a threat to the whole office's existence.

Such boundaries between different sex workers were sometimes managed through the organization of space. In one drop-in center I often visited, a room marked off by a curtain separated women who slept in the office regularly after doing sex work from the peer educators and outreach workers coming in to fill out paperwork or attend meetings. At the time of my field-work, Daisy, a young woman who drank often and wore torn, deep-necked tops, spent time primarily in the rest room during the day and did sex work near bus stands at night. When Daisy came out of the rest room, people often fell silent and looked away: her presence marked a sharp contrast to the other women. After a round of board elections, I asked Indira, one of the elected leaders, why Daisy had not run for office, since she had been coming to the office for so many years. "We thought it's better for those people not to," she said vaguely. Over time, Daisy had become increasingly bitter. "Do you know what kind of people they are? They pretend," she told me, when we finally sat for an interview. "They say if you have money you run the world, right? . . . If you don't have money, stay away from here [this office]." According to her, all the office staff cared about was how much money you had—not really helping one another. A year after I first met her, Daisy had disappeared; when I asked about her, I was told she was gone without further explanation.

Daisy had, in other words, threatened the caste and class respectability the CBO office members prized. Others learned to adapt their modes of engaging with others to fit in with office practice. Mala, for example, a CBO leader, had once been a self-described rowdy who bullied other street sex workers. She told me she had begun working at her first HIV prevention NGO as a way of having a respectable office she could tell her family about, while she continued sex work on the side. But working with NGOs had taught her to be more smooth, to know "how to talk in the right way to the right people." In the beginning, she recalled, "I said, you want a [funding] proposal? Give me a white sheet, and I'll write down the proposal for you right now. I didn't know a proposal was this thick . . . ! Now they've got my hands tied," she said. As she moved around the city for her work, her body had changed too: "I was even fatter then. If I went around my legs would become red. I couldn't walk. I was very fat, and I would sweat from the heat. I always had a box of powder with me." In conversations at the office, Mala would often tell me how rough she had once been. "Ask them how I used to be," she'd say, pointing to the women around us, and they would laugh and nod. Asha, another CBO leader, told me in an interview:

> Our Mala was very rough. If we saw her coming, we'd all hide. But today she has changed a lot . . . about whom to talk to, how to talk to whom, how to be with whom. She has changed. [The CBO] has changed a lot also, I feel. She used to talk so much then. Because she has changed, all the other women have changed too. Even me. I was a big fighter before. Whoever I came across, I'd be drinking and hitting them first thing; that's all I did. Now I know the way to speak to whom, how to work, what time to do what work, and how to make plans. I've changed in the CBO. I didn't know anything before. I didn't even know how to read the bus number. Today I can look at that bus number and read what town the bus is going to. After I came here, I learned all those things.

Inspired by Mala, Asha had learned to navigate public space on the bus, to follow office timings, to talk to people, and to plan ahead. Like Mala, she was no longer rough.

These accounts of gendered embodiment—Preethi's soft voice on the bus, Aparna's neatness, Mala's gentler way of speaking, and Daisy's refusal to change the way she dressed—conformed to a relatively similar view of what it meant to be respectable in public: a middle-class, dominant-caste ideal of modest clothing, modest speech, nonconfrontational behavior, gentleness, and control of bodily desires over roughness, physical excess, and lust.[12] As I have suggested, though, respectability didn't always look the same to all the HIV prevention workers I met. What it meant to behave respectably also became a subject of debate. Once, at an HIV prevention drop-in center, an encounter between Akshay, a working-class kothi, and Shobana, an upwardly mobile transgender woman who had big dreams to become an Indian Administrative Service (IAS) officer, crystallized tensions about what it meant to be respectably feminine. Shobana did not dress like other transgender women at the office. Rather than wearing sparkly *salwar kameezes* and saris and flashy jewelry, Shobana usually wore a T-shirt and jeans, like other middle-class Bangalore law students. She often spoke in English, which infuriated Akshay. Akshay, a kothi, always dressed in plain pants and shirt and identified strongly as working class. He avoided any behavior or language that would out him in public spaces. He often complained about rich, English-speaking gay men he had met and their arrogance, and he was suspicious of anyone tossing English around at the office, too. Once, as Shobana and I sat drinking tea and talking, Akshay joined in. Akshay looked at Shobana. "I always tell her," he said, "if you could only wear some nice earrings and a bindi, you would look so nice. You're always saying people get confused about you." I asked Shobana what Akshay meant by confused. Shobana explained, "Sometimes people don't know when I'm walking around if I'm male or female. If I dressed the way he says, in a sari, people would know." Shobana was wearing jeans and a T-shirt, no jewelry, no makeup, and her shoulder length hair loose." This is my choice," she said. "I also don't wear those things," I said. "At least you're wearing a bindi and earrings and a nose ring," Akshay said. "And I hope you don't mind my saying, but you would look even better if you wore bangles and toe rings! It's how an Indian woman (*bhāratiya nāri*) should look. It looks nice. If you're always saying you're female, you should dress like it!" "There are lots of ways to be a bhāratiya nāri," I said. Shobana agreed. "This is also a way of being Indian," she said. "But why do you have to dress like this?" Akshay insisted, now appealing to both of us. "Don't feel bad," said Shobana, after he left in a bit of a huff. "He's just joking," I said. Shobana agreed but added, "He's a little joking and a little serious." He came back a little while later. "You're always talking in English, or Tamil," he complained to Shobana. "You're so haughty," he added switching to English. "You . . . bastard!" He said that in English too. "Did you hear that? He said bastard!" said Shobana, now offended. "That is a bad word. I have to tell him." Later, she approached Akshay. "You can't say all these rough words," she admonished. "If you do, I'll put an agenda on you!"[13]

Shobana's aspirations for educated, middle-class, modern femininity came into conflict with Akshay's more traditional image of the working-class bhāratiya nāri with toe rings and bangles. To him, Shobana's style was not respectable, not even legible as feminine; to her, it was crucial to her social mobility. As Akshay's outburst revealed the cracks in his own respectability, Shobana warned him not to become rough. Meanwhile, Akshay pointed to class hierarchies and inequalities, mocking Shobana's English-speaking affectations and middle-class jeans. The office, a shared space for these kinds of conflicts, thus became a venue in which embodiments of respectability, and class and caste hierarchies, could be practiced and contested, broken and reinforced.

Respectable embodiment made it possible to navigate public space, often by blending in. But blending in coexisted with an additional skill: opening up about sexual matters in the right contexts.[14] While different organizations held different positions on the question of how open members would ideally be, all the organizations I studied expected members to be comfortable talking about their sexual lives in some contexts. Shanti, a transgender woman who had started out as an HIV prevention worker and moved into human rights activism, called this new quality a *claimingness*. "Ten years ago," she said, "not a single person was coming very openly . . . to claim their identity that I am a transgender, I am a homosexual, I am a bisexual, I am a lesbian. . . . But now, that kind of claimingness has come forward."

The claimingness, or openness, Shanti described was shaped by forces beyond the spaces of HIV prevention, and at least partly it resulted from the broader consolidation of queer visibility and activism in India. But openness was, nevertheless, a relatively new practice for most of my interviewees when they first became involved with HIV prevention. Mostly poor and working-class, my interviewees had been involved in various forms of communal life with other sex workers, sexual minorities, and transgender people before becoming involved in HIV prevention programs, but they had typically not participated in political activism or formal organization on that basis. Openness formed part of the mandate of the National AIDS Control Program, and an organization called the Center for Advocacy and Research (CFAR) was tasked, in part, with training people to practice it. Isaac, who worked for CFAR at the time of my fieldwork, explained,

> Our main job was to make them open. Slowly. We had initial tactics, like, we said give your voice, but you don't need to show your face, you don't need to tell your name. . . . So they started coming to the media and talking, without a name, and without a face. But in three years, with some pioneers . . . in every district we had at least four or five people . . . . we started providing them capacity building. . . . When you talk to the media, don't talk like a grandmother (*ajji*). Only answer to the point. Don't cry. If you don't want to talk, say no comment. . . . we trained them.

As openness was so consciously promoted in HIV prevention programs, in what the anthropologist Adia Benton calls "the imperative to talk,"[15] many described their first encounter with openness as one of the most jarring elements of their first visit to an HIV prevention drop-in center. Neema, for example, had been afraid the first few times she had visited the office and was unsure of what to say. Then, she said, "everyone was saying 'I am also a sex worker,' this and that, so I opened up in front of everyone and talked. . . . I found out that in counseling, we can say what's in our mind. I didn't used to tell anyone. . . . whatever it is you can say it here." Sheela had a similar experience, at a more activist-oriented organization. "When I went to a protest against ITPA, I came to know this word called *sex worker*. I understood that if I identified myself as a sex worker it would be easy to identify other sex workers, and if I didn't it would be difficult. . . . If I hide my identity then you will hide, too. I now announce openly, no problem, though I have not said it on TV yet. I said it while wearing a burqa at a public function." Openness was key to both the work of HIV prevention and to the work of activism, though both Neema and Sheela indicate the negotiations they had to make in order to embrace it. Neema's decision to identify as a sex worker, but only while wearing a burqa, allowed her to embrace openness while protecting her respectability.

Openness was often, at first, an uncomfortable proposition. Priya described her first experience at an HIV prevention CBO. She, like Neema, had been scared:

The other women talked about how clients took off their clothes and did sex for a whole hour, and all that. I was disgusted that they used such filthy words. . . . One of them asked me how many times I had done sex work that day. I was taken aback by her direct question. She told me that all the women did the same work there. . . . They told me to answer with my eyes open. They asked me if I had undressed or if I had done sex wearing all my clothes. . . . I understood that in the office, we had to say everything. . . . When they asked me how many times I did it, I would show my hand to say once, twice, or four times. They told me not to show my hand but to tell them. . . . The other women would laugh when I showed my hand like that, saying it looked like I was giving a benediction.

Priya had learned to be open against her initial inclinations, slowly growing more comfortable speaking about her life as a sex worker. "I was a fool," she said, reflecting on her early days.

The office itself provided a crucial site for practicing openness. One office I visited, of a CBO for women in sex work, sat on a major street but was simultaneously hidden. It was surrounded by construction, at the top of a narrow, dark staircase, so its bright, airy layout and shiny marble floors came as a surprise. Posters lined the walls, and the office was full of natural light. I was told Bill Gates, the South African minister of health, and the director of NACO had visited this office, along with a couple of film stars—Kamal Hassan and Vasundhara Das. None of this was clear from the street, where not even a sign marked the office. Once in the office, as members opened up, the office became an intimate space for sharing what many of my interviewees called their *kaṣṭa-sukha*, their difficulties and happinesses, their ups and downs. I was often told that being open made it possible for others to be open—if you shared your kaṣṭa-sukha, others would feel comfortable sharing theirs. In this way, openness laid the groundwork for friendship and care,[16] even if it also involved risk. Openness was carefully calibrated for different moments, safe within the office but not always without. Vandana, an HIV prevention worker at a CBO, began telling me in an interview about how she had once felt ashamed about being a sex worker but had learned to feel less so as she learned how many others like her there were. I asked if she still felt ashamed. "There's nothing to be ashamed about. Why be ashamed at being a sex worker? But you just can't say it with outside people, that's all. I can say it to people here [in the CBO], people who are like me." Mala put it more bluntly: "Look, I don't eat all the time. I eat when I'm hungry. Like that, I don't just tell everyone I'm a sex worker. At a place when I need to, I say it."

Outside of the office setting, for even the most seasoned activists and HIV prevention workers, openness about sex work, sexual identity, or HIV status was a fraught personal challenge. Only a few of my interviewees, for example, had told their whole families they did sex work; a few more had told one or two trusted family members later in life. Some cisgender women planned to tell their families after their children were married, so as not to endanger marriage prospects, but others avoided the issue completely. Those who did disclose almost always had broken contact with some members of their families. For transgender women, who had often already contended with disclosure when they left home, openness was easier, but still often selective. Those who did sex work still often left that part out of family conversations.

And yet, openness was often debated and held up as a standard within HIV prevention and activist spaces. Lata, for example, a long-time sex worker activist, told me emphatically that she hoped more sex workers would "stand openly": "The day you leave your shyness behind and come out, that's the day you'll live well," she said. Yet one day, Lata told me how upset she was that someone had accused her of not opening up and identifying as a sex worker. "I do say it! I always say it. You've heard it, haven't you?" she insisted. Another time, I attended a meeting of AIDS activists in Bangalore, at which one of the participants, Suchitra, said she had chosen not to speak about being positive with her family. Shankar, an NGO worker at the meeting, urged, "If after thirteen years of being positive, you still don't tell your family, even though you're so healthy . . . what are you going to go tell anyone else?" Suchitra shot back, "And then my brother's daughter has to get married." Shankar continued to push. "Can't you tell them if you can tell everyone else? What do you want, your family, or this work?" Suchitra held her ground. "I want both!" she exclaimed. "Don't talk about this, Shankar," another participant intervened. "Let's change the topic."

A week later, when I asked Shankar if he thought openness was a necessity for activism around sexuality, he was more measured: "When sex workers demand their rights, when that kind of environment is created, definitely the collective can raise their voice, but on the individual level, we cannot force. . . . we don't know the consequences of that. What could happen to them? They could be distanced from their families, they could be put out of their house, their child's education could be discontinued. When those kind of things happen, who will be responsible?" Openness was valued and contested in HIV prevention spaces. One talked about sexuality both for the purposes of HIV prevention and for the purposes of political activism. But very few actually applied this principle in all realms of life, and the ability to be open when necessary and blend in when it wasn't was a skill many cultivated as part of their HIV prevention work. This selective openness made it possible to make identity-based political demands and to conduct HIV outreach, without endangering norms of respectability and discretion.[17]

What it meant to be a selectively open, respectable and confident target of HIV prevention was never stable. How open to be, or what it meant to look and behave respectably, was up for debate. HIV prevention programs did not foreclose or impose a single way of inhabiting these norms. What they did do, however, was provide an environment in which norms could be learned, practiced, and even argued over.

"HIV GAVE ME AN IDENTITY"

Many of my interviewees told me that the AIDS response formed a platform or a catalyst for sex worker, sexual minority, and transgender activism. As Raghu, an activist and NGO director, put it, "HIV gave me an identity. It got people out of the closet. It brought the community out into the open." Raghu implied that the virus itself was the basis of identity claims, that sexual identity was premised on being a subject of HIV prevention. In practice, this process of being "given an identity" through HIV took place through three mechanisms: naming practices, diversified income, and shared space.

The naming and classification practices of HIV prevention programs across India have been widely critiqued, from both within and outside the HIV industry, for imposing unnecessary boundaries, for rendering certain noncategorizable subjects illegible, for misgendering transgender people, and for imposing biomedical categories on complex and fluid social experiences, among other issues.[18] Despite often heated debates, naming practices continued to be central to the everyday experience of the HIV prevention workers and activists I interviewed. Part of joining a CBO, many interviewees told me, was learning how to name yourself.

HIV prevention programs initially used three strict categories for high-risk groups—men who have sex with men (MSM), female sex worker (FSW), and IV drug user (IDU)—and funded separate organizations for each group. Later iterations of sexual health programming, such as the Pehchan Project, or Recognition Project, developed the category of MSM-TG-Hijra (MTH).[19] Categorizations like kothi, *satla-kothi*, double-decker, *panthi*, bisexual, and *jogappa* were also used to categorize MSMs in the KSAPS and KHPT documents I reviewed.[20] FSWs were less often described as an internally differentiated group, but their sites of solicitation—brothel-based, street-based, home-based, etc.—were categorized and documented.

Regardless of the specific language used, knowing the category one belonged to was central to the process of becoming an HIV prevention worker and to everyday practice within HIV offices. The Sunday meeting of one CBO I often visited always began with a round of introductions: My name is _____, and I'm a _____, each person would say, and these same introductions would be used when members attended outside events, trainings, or political rallies. Once, I arrived at the office to find two visiting students from Sweden, dressed in the kind of baggy tie-dye pants and T-shirts I only ever saw on European tourists. Geetika, the program manager of the office, asked me to translate as everyone in the office gathered in a circle. We went around in a circle to do introductions. Everyone said what part of Karnataka they were from, which I didn't translate, and their sexual identity. One person identified as a DD, and I explained that this stood for double-decker. The students asked what that meant, and Geetika said we could wait till later to explain. At the end of the introductions, we explained DD— "someone who likes to do sex and have sex done to them," Geetika said. Learning how to describe one's identity, using correct terms, and explain it to others was an important part of initiation. Srinivas, for example, who worked at another CBO, told me warily of new members who lacked clarity about who they were: "Many people don't know. Am I a kothi, TG, DD, bisexual? They need to have clarity about [the question of] what I am. I should know I'm a bisexual. They are confused. [Why is this important?] They are confused. Some say I'm a panthi. They'll be DD, but they'll say they're panthi. They don't know with clarity. They should be able to say it themselves. . . . . [Were you also that way?] I was confused. I'd say, why do you call me kothi? After training, I understood. Now, I say I'm bisexual." Such an account of learning to describe one's identity correctly, after appropriate training, was almost universal among those I interviewed. Satya, who identified himself as a double-decker, explained that, after a training session, he found out "that there was a name[21] for what I do." At times, naming oneself seemed like a precondition of participation in HIV prevention spaces. In his book about the Gates Foundation's Avahan program, its former director Ashok Alexander tells of a moment when a transgender woman approached Bill Gates while he was on a site visit. Touching his feet in a sign of respect, she whispered, "TG" (transgender).[22]

These practices within HIV prevention spaces did not mean epidemiological terms were all-encompassing. Many interviewees recognized that the more rigid conventions around naming they developed in HIV prevention drop-in centers were distinct from the more fluid usages they might use in other contexts. Malini, a transgender woman, described the first time she realized that the grand-sounding phrase *sex work* really just described what she already did every night: "Here [in the office] these people speak English; they say I do sex, sex work. Actually when I first heard [the term] *sex work*, I had thought it must be some other job!. . . . One time, wondering what job someone went for, when I went with him for sex work, I realized that he goes to [the bus stand] Majestic. . . . I said, 'I did this too last night! Is this what *sex work* is?'" While naming was central to being part of an HIV prevention CBO, Malini's skepticism points to the fact that many members recognized the limits of naming even as they regularly engaged in it. On the one hand, for example, Lakshman embraced the name *kothi*:

> Normally if someone asks my gender or sexuality, I say I'm a homosexual kothi, but if you say, do you do sex work, I'll say, yes, I'm a sex worker. [Where did you first hear this concept?] When I came to the organization, [I learned] oh, it's like this, there are these categories and this language, and I can be like this and tie my hair. In society I'm [seen as] a boy, right? I used to mingle with hijras personally, but I didn't know I was a kothi like this. When that question came about sexuality, when they said it's called *kothi*, then I learned what *sex work* and *sexuality* mean, and how many people there are like me.

Yet Lakshman was simultaneously critical of HIV prevention funding for its rigidity of categories. "KSAPS keeps MSM, transgender, and hijra separate. . . . I'm an MSM, but tomorrow I wear a sari and get a blood test, and then if I get an operation I'm a hijra, then I'm a transgender. However I identify, they should recognize it. Why keep them separate?" It was clear to Lakshman that naming was central to his path into the CBO but also that it belied the fluidity of practice.

Naming, as Lakshman's own complex position suggests, was the site of contestation within the hybrid spaces of HIV prevention, and categories were negotiated, challenged, and reworked. Naming circulated from HIV prevention NGOs and helped solidify class and caste hierarchies within communities of sex workers, sexual minorities, and transgender people, encapsulated in access to the English language. As activists Sunil Mohan and Rumi Harish write, "due to the increasing dominance of NGOs . . . many new English identities and words now circulate around India and are picked up by our communities . . . Funding politics and NGOs play a major role in bringing the caste, class and religion based politics of understanding the names and where they belong."[23] Hari, for example, said he identified sometimes as kothi, sometimes as double-decker. "Why should I say a particular identity? What I feel now is genderless. . . . Why should I say this is my identity? Why should that be fixed? I don't want it fixed, I want it flexible."

Another mechanism by which HIV prevention programs could be the site for reinvention was the diversification of income. Hari had become involved in HIV prevention work in the early 2000s and had learned a variety of skills—conducting outreach, documenting sexual behavior, and writing grants. He was even forming a new NGO of his own. When he reflected on his previous life, when he had done sex work, he explained, "I was rough then. The way I used to talk. Now if people see me, they think I've become smooth. My old friends tell me I've changed so much." He elaborated:

> When doing sex work, I had some moments when I was very happy. I enjoyed spending time near the Vidhana Soudha till midnight, waiting for clients, and when we didn't get clients, joking with the community, and joking with the police. There were some good moments like that, but there were also bad experiences, like *gūṇḍās* [goons] coming and scaring us and stealing things, proposing sex, and police demanding money, and when we had no money, saying they would file cases, and demanding sex too. I faced all that. Sometimes when sex work didn't happen, I couldn't go home, and where could I go? I'd wander in the bus stop. Then I was introduced to [the NGO.] When I had clients I did sex work, and when I

didn't I went to rallies and protests, gave information to the community, and attended Sunday meetings. . . . I started full-time [NGO] work. I decreased sex work a lot. Not that I oppose sex work, but I felt that I didn't want it for me, so I didn't do it.

In the process of "becoming smooth," Hari had learned to occupy NGO spaces. He had learned to facilitate meetings with foreign visitors and community members, to write a proposal or report for a funder, and to do fieldwork, meeting community members in the field. Sex work had been, for him, neither solely dangerous and undesirable nor solely fun and liberating. Nevertheless, NGO work had increasingly come to replace sex work as a source of income.

Radha, an HIV outreach worker, described a similar trajectory away from sex work as she became involved in HIV prevention. Radha was the main earner in her family and was plagued by debt. She had worked as a manual laborer and domestic laborer when she first exchanged sex for money. She had continued to do sex work, and later took up a job as a housekeeper, but after a bad traffic accident, she was unable to continue. Now once more without a steady source of income, Radha found HIV prevention work. She took out a ₹4000 loan, with which her son bought a cow, eventually paying for his sister's wedding and a new house. After seven years in HIV prevention, Radha was an outreach worker, continued to do sex work, and also had eight cows. Both her children were married, she had a house, and she had even paid for a leg operation. "If [the CBO] hadn't opened, I wouldn't have come to this level," she said.

While not all organizations provided loans, as Radha's did, the steady income HIV prevention work provided offered an important supplement to more unpredictable sex work income, and meant reducing the amount of time a member spent on sex work each day. This diversified income meant sex work figured less prominently in their everyday lives, and made soliciting the same number of clients every day a less urgent necessity. Diversified income meant HIV prevention workers had more control over when they did sex work and how openly they went about it.

Anchoring these pedagogies of naming and this diversification of income was a specific spatial context: the HIV prevention drop-in center. The geographer Phil Hubbard argues that the spatial restriction of "bad citizens" who challenge heteronormativity can paradoxically create "sex zones" that become sites of experimentation and liberation, and forms of citizenship that allow both public claims and privacy.[24] Like the gay and lesbian villages Hubbard talks about, HIV prevention offices became sites for self-making and friendship. Walk up the stairs to one of the "MSM CBO" offices I often visited, and you would be greeted first by a pile of shoes. Once they crossed the threshold of the office, people moved their bodies more fluidly; the boundaries between bodies seemed less rigid, people snuggled or played with each other's hair, rested their heads on one another's laps or shoulders, and joked or argued for hours on end. Music might be on. On some days, the space became an impromptu dance party, and the sharpest dancers had their moment to shine. People would stop in when passing by to see who was around and say hello; sometimes, more formal visitors—researchers, groups of social work students, KSAPS officers, or even health officials from other states or countries—would arrive for more formal introductions to the organization's work. If you came in the late morning or the early afternoon, the air in the office filled with the fragrance of tea. Everyone knew this tea was the best: milky, thick, and boiled for long enough to be rich and sweet. Nearing six, people would start getting ready to leave, crowding around the mirror near the door as they applied a new coat of powder or lipstick before going together to do sex work.

The offices I visited varied in how they were organized. Most had posters bearing hand-drawn maps of the nearby "hot-spots" hung on the wall, along with the more generic HIV prevention posters. Most had a television somewhere and piles of the ubiquitous cardboard boxes of Nirodh (government-brand) condoms crammed in a corner. Some had an area with Hindu idols for small rituals (*pūjās*), evoking an air of respectable Hindu domesticity. "It's like your mother's house," people would often tell me. In some offices, people seemed focused on paperwork; in others, people rarely seemed to be doing anything related to HIV prevention. Across organizations, though, the physical space of the office offered respite from the potentially brutal experience of being a sex worker, sexual minority, or transgender person on the street. These were intimate spaces, warm and sometimes raucous. They were spaces where the boundaries of respectability could be learned and contested. They were also spaces where openness about sexuality could be embodied indoors and in daylight—rather than outdoors, at night, in hidden alleyways and behind trees in public parks. They were spaces in which, even temporarily, criminalized sexualities did not have to take cover in darkness.[25]

In some cases, people used the office to conduct sex work indoors, away from the threat of police harassment or someone from the village who could pass news on to one's family. One afternoon, for example, I sat in a drop-in center with two cisgender woman sex workers, Soundarya and Sharada, playing carrom. As we played, they passed the phone back and forth to talk to clients. One client called Soundarya, and she passed the phone to her friend, clearly the bolder of the two. "What's the news?" she laughed into the phone. The client asked for an *all round*, and Sharada's eyes grew wide as she mocked him. "What is that?" she asked, incredulous. "Rubbing? You want to rub?" she said loudly, daring him to say it louder. "I'm just not understanding. You want to rub?" Finally, he hung up. "Poor thing, he says he wants to rub or something," she said, laughing to the others. An older woman sat a bit apart from the conversation, watching them carefully, not playing carrom or participating in the banter. Soundarya was talking about some friend who went with a client for five days. "It's five days and he gives ₹20,000," apparently, she said. They talked about it with some dismissiveness. "I'll go," says Puttamma. I don't get anyone these days. Shilpa looked at her. "I tell it like it is, so don't be upset by this," she said. "But if we can't even get clients, what clients will you get?" Puttamma was silent. As these negotiations suggest, the drop-in center became a site for negotiating the terms of sex work. From a safe, private location, sex workers had room to negotiate with clients, share clients, and laugh over unexpected experiences, as well as to compare notes about rates and services. Importantly, this protected location also made it easier to refuse a client. It also, as Puttamma's intervention shows, could be a site for reproducing hierarchies of age, as well as caste and class.

In addition to serving as a space for sharing clients and conferring over prices, an office meant shared space to compare notes on clothes, makeup, and jewelry. Once, for example, I bought Geetika a *dupatta* after she had told me she had been looking for one like what I was wearing and couldn't find one anywhere. Geetika looked pleased as she untwisted it. "How much was it?" Amisha asked, walking over to inspect it. When I told her, I caught a flicker of judgment in her eyes at my bargaining skills, but then she smiled generously. "But you have to look at the quality," she said, and I wondered if she meant it. "Don't iron it," Amisha advised Geetika. "That's the style." In an interview, Lekha described how she had learned to dress once she became an HIV peer educator: "I used to wear very rural clothes; that's how they raised me at home. . . . if you do sex you can't dress like that. So I stopped dressing like a village girl. As much of a village girl I was, I would wear makeup like a town girl. . . . Now [at the CBO] all the girls wear flowers, wear bangles . . . and now joining with them, now I do all this. . . . After I came to [the CBO] I learned how to dress." Sometimes, instruction in how to behave and dress respectably was more explicit. Paralleling Lekha's journey away from the embodiment of a "village girl" to that of a "town girl" and then back to a more traditional look, Pallavi described how she learned to manage her voice:

> I got courage from attending the meetings here. I learned how to talk to different kinds of people and the way to approach different kinds of people in different situations. We are rural people, and earlier I would speak crudely. . . . In Bangalore one should talk neatly, prettily, with discipline. The words that come out of my mouth should not hurt anybody. I have been shouted at a lot in this office. They used to say that I had not learned anything even after so many years, and that I talked strangely. Now I have become perfect. I can go to any person and talk to him without fear. They praise me now.

Pallavi's account captures the balance of discipline and boldness, respectability and openness. She had been taught to "talk neatly," and this new skill allowed her to talk to anyone "without fear." She had learned the discipline to navigate public space, the forms of behavior that allowed her to blend in, and thus the basis to speak up when she needed.

As a site for experimenting with forms of speech and clothing, the office had the potential to open up new gendered possibilities. For Lavanya, a transgender woman, it had meant learning to embody what she considered a more middle-class, feminine style she contrasted to that of hijras:

> Since I joined as staff, my behavior, activities, and communication with community is completely different. How do you have to talk, and in what way. Because if you look at some of our hijras, they don't talk well. They have very bad behavior, the way they do things, the way they talk, the way they walk, the style . . . but I'm not like that. I talk in a feminine way, and go everywhere decently in a feminine way, and I've learned to sit down as a woman and walk like a woman in every way. I've learned communication in the organization.

For Lavanya, these gradual transformations meant she had the potential to work in the mainstream, to be "in society"—indeed, in the years after I met her, she had moved on to working in a corporate job. Malini, also a transgender woman, felt more regret around the journey she had taken to becoming more gender-conforming. Before, she said, "I wasn't on this side or that side"; she was a "girl in my mind;" and she wore pants and a shirt and wore her hair long. Now, "I have breasts. . . . When someone first looks at me, they think I am a girl. . . . they don't do any ragging or anything. . . . They talk to me like they talk to a girl." The office had partly made this possible: "It's only after coming to this office that I've learned everything new. I didn't even know how to leave my hair [loose]. I didn't know how to pierce my ears. This kind of anklet, toe rings . . . I didn't know even the small things. Now that I've joined with them . . . every day they're doing things like this, putting nail polish. . . . If this office hadn't been there, I wouldn't have become like this. That's what I think. Really." But Malini was critical of these developments:

> I have to say, they should shut down these offices now. . . . It's not good. . . . If they want, let the government put some condom boxes in the bathrooms and go. . . . [Community members] come and don't know what it is. . . . Then they come for one week, they come two weeks, and in the third week they come wearing nail polish. Did they come the fourth week? They'll be wearing bangles on their hands. Then did they come the fifth week? They'll be wearing flowers [in their hair]. . . . by two months, they'll come wearing a sari. If there wasn't an office, many people wouldn't have become like this at all.

For Lavanya, joining an organization had helped her cultivate a new feminine embodiment and opened up possibilities for assimilation and the middle-class job she dreamed of. Malini, meanwhile, insisted she had been "ruined." But both Malini and Lavanya pointed to how the office became a site in which they could take risks with how they looked and experiment with imagining and embodying gender differently.

BECOMING SMOOTH

Two years after I finished the bulk of my fieldwork, Preethi had moved away from HIV prevention work. She continued to live in her own apartment. Her neighbors had become her main support network, a group of women who came by giggling to see me, commenting on the weight I had gained or lost. Preethi no longer went to the CBO office and had left her job in HIV prevention, where, she said, there were no funds. She had completely stopped soliciting on the street and instead spent a week out of a month at a *mane* [house, in this case a brothel] on the edge of Bangalore, where she saw ten to twelve clients a day. She could make enough money that way to pay rent and live comfortably for the rest of the month, supplementing her income with a few long-time clients who called her once in a while. Five years after I first met her, Preethi showed me her employment letter for a new job working as a government clerk. She still had some clients, and she was exploring a new relationship with someone she'd met at her job. She had also received some job training from an NGO working with transgender women. A few days after I saw her, I clicked on a video on Facebook that showed her talking about her employment goals. "I want to work in the mainstream," she told the camera, talking easily and comfortably about the problems faced by transgender people as they searched for employment outside the community. The video showed her dressed in a high-necked, collared, cotton *salwar kameez*, sitting at a computer.

From an activist perspective, these new skills, confidence, and comfort in navigating state institutions were a key outcome of AIDS programs. One NGO director I interviewed noted, "You never heard voices of sex workers and MSMs. They were not in other programs. So yes, there has been tremendous community mobilization. How would you define that? You know, doing stuff for themselves, and being able to take stands. And taking care of each other, sex worker groups taking care of each other in the community. This never happened earlier. Now women are sitting in the planning commission and talking. That never happened earlier. HIV has made that happen." In the years after my fieldwork, I saw many of those I had come to know move out of HIV prevention work. Some moved back into sex work, domestic work, or factory work; some stayed part of the NGO and activist world; and some stayed connected to both. Yet as HIV prevention programs had faded from prominence, there were shifts. Preethi had made herself more respectably feminine even as she had developed confidence advocating for herself as a transgender woman. Naming practices and diversified income, all cultivated in a shared office space in which norms could be practiced and contested, helped create the conditions for Preethi's transformation.

This process was not solely an imposition of a Western or global sexual identity.[26] Rather, the norms of the ideal HIV prevention target were contested and argued over as each participant embarked on a project of developing (or rejecting) the norms of HIV prevention. HIV prevention programs thus provided a shared platform within which sex workers, sexual minorities, and transgender people could cultivate smoother selves. It was not a coercive process but one in which people like Preethi actively worked to change. Tracing Preethi's path offers a way of thinking about how marginalized people engage the state not by resisting or collaborating with it but rather by "using the system as best they can" to secure material stability and even social mobility.[27] While a range of scholars and commentators have noted how AIDS paradoxically catalyzed transformative changes for sex workers in particular,[28] this chapter has demonstrated the intimate processes through which these transformations took place.

India's AIDS crisis was produced within a global AIDS field. The negotiations I have analyzed so far highlight the wide variation in how individuals and organizations navigated the programs the crisis occasioned and how they reinvented sexuality and citizenship within the hybrid spaces the crisis created. But this complexity was often lost in the accounts of India's AIDS programs I read in public health journals or news articles that circulated transnationally. In the 2010s, as the urgency of the AIDS crisis increasingly began to lapse, donors began to move on to new issues and places. In the process, researchers quantified and assessed the Indian AIDS response. In the next chapter I turn to how donors and state agencies represented the complexities of the Indian AIDS response and circulated them in the global AIDS field.

6 | MAKING IT COUNT

EVERY HIV PREVENTION DROP-IN CENTER I visited had a counseling room available for one-on-one consultations. In October 2012, I visited one of these counseling rooms for the first time. A CBO member took me into the counseling area, where a young woman, the counselor in the office, was talking with a new member. The new member had come with a friend who was a peer educator. The counselor was asking a series of questions. In between, she added information about HIV prevention and the CBO's services in a detached, repetitive tone, as though she were listing state capitals or train times. She looked mostly at the questionnaire sheets in front of her and took notes there, glancing up occasionally at the nervous new member and her friend.

At the very first question, the woman's Kannada faltered. "I don't speak Kannada," she said in Hindi. The meeting, somehow, proceeded in Kannada anyway. She sat hunched over in her seat. "There are four ways to get HIV," said the counselor, in a mechanical voice. She listed the ways, without pauses. "Here at the CBO, you could get tested, get loans, and there is a crisis support system." She began filling out the questionnaire. "What do you do?" "I work at a beauty parlor." "How often do you do sex work?" "About twice a month." "How long have you been doing it?" "Do I have to answer?" The new member paused. Her friend had just come into the room. I stepped out, worried about making the encounter even more uncomfortable. "Ten years," I finally heard her say as I left the room.[1]

HIV prevention drop-in centers, as Chapter 5 showed, are important sites for categorizing, naming, and contesting categories of identity and practice, and an experience like this often defines one's first encounter with them. As they spent more time in contact with HIV prevention outreach, sex workers, sexual minorities, and transgender people became more familiar with the process of documenting their experiences. These encounters were expected to take place on a regular basis, both in the office and in the field. Overall, national guidelines stipulated that one peer educator was responsible for maintaining sixty contacts, meeting all of them every week or every other week to document their activity and provide them with condoms.[2]

These monitoring exercises were driven by an HIV prevention program's effort to, as the 2007 national guidelines put it, "improve its quality and achieve its goals."[3] For example, measuring how many condoms a peer educator needed—by multiplying the number of sex workers in an area, the number of sex acts a day, and the number of days a sex worker is active in a month, and subtracting condoms from other sources—ensured condom provision was efficient and eliminated condom dumping or shortages.[4] In aggregate, numbers also served an external function: they enumerated and affirmed India's successful response and made it a model, or best practice. By the time I began my fieldwork in 2012, the Indian AIDS response was considered a success within the global AIDS field. The components of this success were variable and extended beyond the typical elements of a public health program. Within the hybrid spaces of HIV prevention, sex worker, sexual minority, and transgender groups worked on a range of issues, from assisting transgender women who had been detained by police to supporting cisgender women sex workers in getting their children into school. In order for these diverse engagements to count as a success transnationally, they had to be quantified.

This chapter takes up this process of quantification. It highlights how numbers helped solidify a model of HIV prevention that was substantively different from the political engagements this book has analyzed thus far. I argue that quantification was key to repackaging the Indian AIDS response as a model that could be scaled up and circulated in the global AIDS field.

THEY NEED TO TAKE THE MODEL & BRING IT ELSEWHERE

India's AIDS response resulted from a political process, as the state began with a logic of containing sexual deviance and disease, responded to sustained activism by sex workers and sexual minority groups, and navigated relationships with multiple transnational donors. But, as researchers and donors began to quantify the Indian AIDS response, it was reframed not as a political process but as a response to data.[5] This model began with mapping to understand where the AIDS epidemic was concentrated and then providing an intervention package for those populations.[6] Quantitative representations of HIV prevention interventions largely cut out the roles of the state and social movements, which were central to the Indian AIDS response. AIDS in India was thus disentangled from sexual politics. Quantification helped make this possible.

Quantification—or "the use of numbers to describe social phenomena in countable and commensurable terms"[7]—has become increasingly central to how global institutions manage problems, including crisis. Quantification bundles information, confers objectivity, and creates categories of knowledge. Anthropologist Sally Engle Merry shows that indicator culture is increasingly dominant in global governance institutions. She warns that the makers of indicators often "create the world they are measuring."[8] Numbers are key to how global governance institutions measure and compare nation-states to each other as they seek out and evaluate the best models for intervention. Accordingly, quantification forms a central part of the AIDS response—in measuring epidemic patterns, planning responses, and documenting and identifying failures and successes. Rates of infection and evaluations of interventions, once quantified, can travel more easily across geographic boundaries.[9] Even the most basic AIDS estimates have often been subject to fraught debates, false starts, and unexpected recalculations. The celebrated economist Amartya Sen wrote in 2008 about the Indian AIDS epidemic that "the number game of sizing the affected population has been something of an elephants' burial ground."[10]

The colonial history of quantification helps illuminate its contemporary manifestations. Statistical knowledge was tied to discourses of modernity in colonial governance. Statistics allowed colonial planners to measure and assess India's progress against a universal standard.[11] Numbers allowed for a process of normalizing and packaging systems of social classification, like caste and religious community, in Indian society and abstracted them for colonial management.[12] Quantitative scientific study of sexuality—including elaborate typologies of different types of prostitutes—lay the groundwork for colonial social science.[13] Numbers translated social problems and their management from one context to another.[14] Medical sociologists and anthropologists show how these quantification processes and, increasingly, experimental logics continue to operate as a governance mechanism.[15] The production of indicators allows for the comparison of states.[16] Numbers are always constituted in a political process,[17] but once a number "stabilizes and travels out from its context of production," sociologists Elizabeth Berman and Daniel Hirschman note, "the political and epistemological choices that are so explicit during struggles to establish a number disappear."[18] It was through quantification that messy political processes within crisis responses became the basis for comparing one nation-state to another in the global AIDS field.

Because it is so central to how global governance institutions measure, assess, and compare humanitarian interventions across nation-states, quantification illuminates how transnational arenas like the global AIDS field operate, and why some aspects of circulating models travel farther than others. The production of evaluations, scholarly publications, statistical projections, and surveys helped to abstract the complex realities of HIV prevention programs in India and argue for their relevance to other countries' AIDS programs. This chapter follows the process, beginning with the use of numbers to quantify the participatory practices of CBOs and NGOs. It then shifts the vantage point to Kenya as a way of analyzing the representation of India's AIDS response in the global AIDS field, by tracing how this model was reproduced and adapted in Kenya. In this process, the collection of numbers began to overwhelm other organizational activities,[19] and the sexual politics that shaped the AIDS response in India was largely left out.[20]

The quantitative results of India's AIDS response were notable and impressive. News articles carried the estimate that the Gates Foundation's Avahan initiative had prevented over one hundred thousand HIV infections in India between 2003 and 2008,[21] drawing from a study published in the prestigious medical journal *The Lancet*.[22] "Avahan showed it can be done," wrote James Robertson, the executive director of the India HIV/AIDS Alliance in 2014.[23] Bill Gates, after a visit to a sex worker CBO in Bangalore in 2012, wrote on his blog, "The India program stands out as one of the best examples of effective national scale up of HIV prevention efforts, but those efforts will need sustained funding and government leadership. We're hoping that what we learn in India will encourage and guide increased prevention efforts in other parts of the world."[24]

Gates' interest in "what we learn in India" reflected the link between quantification and its ultimate goal: building an example, or model, that could be circulated transnationally. Monika Krause calls such a model "the good project."[25] Krause argues that donors and humanitarian institutions increasingly work to produce good projects, not necessarily to achieve good outcomes. In line with Krause's analysis, research publications about India's AIDS response, especially those funded by Avahan, talked about success and replicability almost interchangeably. Already in 2006, Avahan documents noted the coming shift toward "packaging the learnings from Avahan."[26] Avahan's evaluations were designed to develop a product: a globally replicable large-scale and cost-effective model for HIV prevention.[27] The definition of success was to build a model, not to sustain a program.[28] "It did not lead to strengthening public health systems," a Bangalore activist told me. "The Gates theory is we are there to stimulate the program; now we've done our job, we are leaving," explained a former NACO official in an interview. The Gates Foundation innovated, tracked its results, and proved a concept, and then shifted to developing models somewhere else. It exemplified the process of quantifying, scaling up, and moving on that has increasingly become an organizing principle of crisis intervention and humanitarian projects.

ENUMERATING PARTICIPATION

One major challenge of quantifying HIV prevention programs was that they focused on issues of empowerment and community solidarity that were difficult to count. Researchers involved in tracking India's AIDS response used several indicators to track participation. The national NGO and CBO Operational Guidelines, for example, used a *log-frame* (short for *logical framework*).[29] Under the larger goal of reducing STI infection to less than 10% in three years, the log frame set a series of objectives with specific indicators attached to each. For example, under the objective of creating an "environment supportive to service delivery and community development," indicators included the number of people who attended street theater productions, the number of police officers who attended orientation programs, and the number of rallies conducted, with the number of participants in each, for

World AIDS Day.[30] Quantification was as central to evaluation as it was to planning and monitoring. For example, a 2012 KHPT study created empowerment variables based on measures such as sex workers' confidence in seeking advice, their comfort in being identified as sex workers, their ability to rely on other sex workers for support, the extent of networks of peers they could trust, and whether they had a bank account and found a statistically significant association between several of the measures and self-efficacy for condom use.[31]

Quantifying the work of community organizations, as sophisticated as the measures were, tended to narrow the scope of what that participation could entail, both on paper and in practice. One example was the elections CBOs conduct every year.[32] I was involved in two such elections at two different CBOs while I was conducting fieldwork. The elections suggested how the production of numbers aimed to affirm the value of participation but also had the immediate effect of orienting organizational work toward the quantity, rather than the character, of participation.

On the day of the election at one of the CBOs, the office buzzed with excitement. Two tables had been set up in the back of the room, each with an electronic voting machine, partitioned off with a booth constructed from used NACO condom boxes (NIRODH LUBRICATED, the boxes said.) "Can I take a picture of you explaining things to people?" one of the staff who had come to visit asked me, looking around at the scene. Discussions ensued about how to make sure the sex workers coming to vote understood how. The previous year, the candidates had chosen graphic symbols, as is done in Indian government elections; this year, tiny, grainy photos of the candidates had been printed for the voting booth, leaving most voters squinting in confusion. The button the voter had to press after voting was another object of concern. If we told voters to push the "yellow" button in English, they might think we were saying the Kannada word *ella* [all], as in "push all the buttons"; if we used the correct Kannada word, *haḷadi*, people may or may not know what it meant. When the first voter arrived, she told me her name was Gangamma. I peered at the list of members the NGO staff had given me. There were some fifteen Gangammas on the list. To narrow it down, I asked her age. She was twenty-six. There was no twenty-six-year-old Gangamma on the list. "Put that one," Gita, one of my election coworkers, advised me, pointing to a Gangamma who was thirty.

Early in the day, most of us were careful about following procedure. As the day progressed and monotony set in, things started to slide. A woman in a bright turquoise sari came in but didn't know what to say when I asked her name and age. "They're asking me all sorts of things," she called out to the outreach worker who had brought her in, standing just outside the voting area. "What should I say?" Finally, she walked out and then walked back in. I asked Gururaj, another volunteer, what had happened. "She had given her name as Jyothi before, but her real name is Latha. She's on the list," he assured me, before taking her into the booth. "Whose name should I say? Mine?" called out another voter to the outreach worker who had brought her as she entered the voting area. "Her age might be wrong on the list; just mark her anyway," another outreach worker said.

As time went on, outreach workers began following more and more women into the voting booth to point out which candidates they should vote for. I stopped one, recalling the election rules on which I had taken diligent notes at the election committee meeting the day before. "But she doesn't know anything!" the outreach worker said to me indignantly. She whispered to the woman the numbers of the candidates to vote for and handed her over to Gururaj, who took her into the booth, guiding her hands to the selected candidates. "She's never come here before! This is her first time!" another outreach worker said when I tried to check a voter against the list. By the early afternoon, word came from one of the organizers that we should keep the polls open later to try to get more voters. The election workers kept sending text messages to their friends in other zones to find out how many people had voted. "How many came in our zone?" they kept asking.

When I tell this story in a US context, people often read it as a cautionary tale of corruption in a place where corruption is rampant. Some sociologists might point to how the goals or cultural expectations of locals are misaligned with those of donors.[33] But my interlocutors would challenge this interpretation. Certainly, using multiple names is a survival strategy many sex workers and other stigmatized people use on a daily basis to protect themselves. But the use of this and other practices of generating numbers sometimes unmoored from reality were not in opposition to AIDS programs' quantification efforts—they resulted from them.

Scholars and activists have written critically about the emphasis on quantitative data in Indian HIV prevention programs, especially in the period after the start of the Gates Foundation's Avahan initiative.[34] Donor expectations prioritized the production of numbers. The report *Chasing Numbers Betraying People* documented the problems of this focus on data-gathering.[35] The high targets that programs gave to their peer educators and community mobilizers meant they were under pressure to bring in large numbers of their peers for HIV testing, with low pay (₹1,500, or US$21, per month), while working often many more hours than their volunteer status implied. In response to these difficult working conditions, peer educators described promising money, food, or even sex to their peers in exchange for getting tested; bringing in friends for multiple tests; or bringing in people who were not part of high-risk groups. For HIV-positive people, confidentiality was sometimes severely compromised as peer educators scrambled to get more tests done quickly.[36] In this context, it was no surprise that a general election in an organization of sex workers had focused more on the quantitative elements of participation than on its substance.

These accounts suggest the uneasy fit between the quantitative focus of state requirements and donor assessments and the participatory practices of grassroots HIV prevention. On the one hand, quantification tended to narrow the focus of CBOs' participatory activities to those that could be measured, and documenting requirements took up considerable time. On the other hand, quantification could affirm the value of such participatory practices, and build evidence for their efficacy, within the global AIDS field. One KHPT official told me, "[In the] initial stage, people who were working in the Gates Foundation, all management specialists who were from McKinsey, they started coming. . . . I'm talking about . . . elections within communities. They were asking me, what the hell are you people doing? Why do you want to go for elections? I used to say you'll realize after five years why we are doing that. . . . I'm able to train thirty thousand sex workers, a huge amount . . . they started realizing that is important. . . . seven years later, now Gates Foundation people take the Karnataka program and talk about only community mobilization." Kumar noted how the value of a community mobilization process that included elections was revealed in the numbers. As HIV prevention programs in Karnataka broadened to include addressing violence and stigma, challenging the legal environment, and developing democratically controlled organizations, quantification went with it. Assessments counted the numbers of positive articles written on sex workers, or the number of times CBOs had intervened in a legal case on behalf of kothis and hijras. This focus extended to elections. It mattered that the election had occurred, that a large number of sex workers had participated, and that the voting process had been managed smoothly and efficiently. It mattered less who participated and how, or the kinds of leadership the CBO cultivated. Quantification did not make participation, empowerment, or community leadership irrelevant to HIV prevention. But it promoted a focus on the form and quantity of participation, not the content.[37]

As the voting came to a close, I asked the election workers why they had decided to break the election rules. They reacted with jokes, until they realized I was serious. "She is making a small thing into a big issue," Dayanand told the others. "This is a tiny little thing. They're not running for prime minister, it's just a little election; how will one vote make a difference?" Dayanand was pointing out that the CBO election was an empty ritual[38] of participation. Ultimately, it didn't matter whom the members voted for or whether they were even members of the organization. All that mattered were the numbers.

BIG MONEY AND BIG DATA

Within Karnataka, the uses of quantitative data expanded during the third National AIDS Control Programme (NACP III), during which Karnataka was a focus state for the Gates Foundation's Avahan initiative. The Gates Foundation helped set the terms for how numbers would be used in planning, implementing, assessing, and circulating information about HIV prevention programs. My interviewees widely agreed that Avahan had intensified monitoring and surveillance.[39] A "data-driven business approach" emphasized "decentralized planning and management" and "saturating target audiences with adequate staff and services, a key feature found in effective advertising."[40] As a Bangalore activist told me, "Avahan started as a market strategy, not a health strategy."

When the Gates Foundation decided to fund an AIDS response in India, it garnered wide attention from the media. As Chapter 2 showed, in the early 2000s, India's AIDS epidemic was considered to be at an early stage, and, within the global AIDS field, it was considered to be the next epicenter of the pandemic, poised to go the way of Africa. One *Times of India* headline announced triumphantly, "Gates Gives India More Than Africa for AIDS."[41] Ashok Alexander, who directed the Avahan program, describes the "jingoism" and "denial" of government officials who believed such a crisis was not imminent. He recounts an early meeting with Bill Gates and the then prime minister Atal Bihari Vajpayee in 2003. "I believe you have been going around spreading alarm," Vajpayee said.[42] Alexander writes that Avahan was the world's largest privately sponsored HIV prevention program.[43]

It is important not to overstate Avahan's role in India's AIDS response, a role which was subject to debate. Some community organizations were wary of Avahan, especially initially. When the Gates Foundation first arrived in India, Avahan funding posed a dilemma to established organizations working with sexual minorities and sex workers. One activist described the conflict her organization faced when deciding whether to accept the funds:

> First I'll tell you why we didn't want to take it and then I'll tell you why we took it. The reasons we didn't want to take it was that we felt that it was too stigmatizing that, you know, the only lens through which sexual minorities were going to be viewed was as diseased people. . . . Second thing we were thinking is that it's very heavy in terms of deliverables. . . .
>
> And then it was very big money in very short time. So we were scared that we would be completely swept into this, and it would overwhelm our agenda. For all these other things were the reasons why we were very reluctant to get into HIV. So for one and a half years we said no, we shouldn't get into it. And also because it was Bill Gates, and corporate money. We were also wary of that. So we know our take on corporatization, and globalization. . . . The reasons why we took it finally were two or three reasons. One was the reality that people were dying. . . . Second thing is, this money gave us the wherewithal and organization to reach out to a whole lot more people. We couldn't have made that kind of reach, if we didn't have this. . . . And also we said that if we don't get into it, we'll become bystanders. You know? The big money will come and it will go to some horrible NGO, and the communities won't be served. We'll become irrelevant. So we have to get in and change the game. So we were very clear that that was the thing. If we are getting in we are not going to compromise on our human rights, social justice issues.

Despite Avahan's scale and reach, and the media attention it got, it mostly built on existing organizational infrastructure. Alexander recalls his experience with Avahan as a slow process of recognizing the limits of his corporate background. "It was dawning on me that my training with McKinsey . . . would not get me very far . . . I had started seeing in these communities a resilience, strength, humour, heroism . . . and it gave me inspiration."[44] Avahan did not actively support advocacy activities or political work by NGOs, but it could not actively discourage them either.[45] One interviewee linked Avahan's successes to existing political culture in India and the strength of activist organizations at the time: "Gandhi could do what he did because you have centuries and centuries of tradition of panchayat, centuries and centuries of tradition of villagers in community-led discussions of how to manage local issues. So it's inevitable that that is how India responds to things. Your Meena Seshus, and VAMPs, and Ashodayas [sex worker organizations and activists]. Avahan built on that. Yes, they brought in an American business model and a model of accountability that was new, but they could only do that because India is open to political collectivization." More established organizations were especially confident about standing up to funders, including Avahan. One activist noted, "For Avahan advocacy was a total anathema. They were like no! Don't do advocacy!. . . . We didn't care because we were there pre-Avahan and we were a strong collective pre-Avahan, so for us it didn't matter. . . . We didn't give them that kind of power or say. We just did what we had to do. . . . By then we were already too powerful." Smaller organizations, however, relied on Avahan for training and funds.

In practice, then, Avahan had a variable role in determining the direction of AIDS programs. But both state officials and activists complained that the Gates Foundation was overstating its role in Indian HIV prevention, presenting itself as an innovator when it was funding the Indian state's ready-made model and the hard work of grassroots community members.[46] One activist I interviewed said Avahan was "only replicating government, not cutting-edge work." A NACO official recalled a shifting relationship between the Gates Foundation and the state: "The initial six months were very good. Gates . . . entirely depended on us for the initial learning process. They acknowledge that mentoring we did for them. Later on, after that, at some point of time, Gates became too big. . . . I used to hear there was a friction between Gates and NACO; Gates was over-projecting themselves. Even though the money they put in was only $200 million, and government money was ten times that, it was almost made to seem as if Gates was running the show."

By 2013, the Gates Foundation's Avahan program was ready to withdraw

WHITE SAVIORISM?

from India.[47] Though the withdrawal had been planned,[48] many of my interviewees saw the exit as a betrayal.[49] "They've ruined everything and they've gone. Who's going to hold them responsible?" asked one interviewee who directed an NGO. "Their project is over, they'll move to Africa, to Kenya, to Tanzania, wherever," noted another activist. J. V. R. Prasada Rao, former director of NACO, now a UNAIDS official, wrote that "the programme, which aimed at ultimate community ownership of the interventions, has initiated the process of transfer before this objective is fully realized."[50] Government officials, NGO workers, and activists alike argued that Avahan had provided substantial funds and received a lot of media airtime but had left behind unsustainable monitoring systems and management costs.[51] For Avahan, meanwhile, its work was complete. Ashok Alexander writes that "Bill was above all a man of science": he saw Avahan's work on prevention and community mobilization as effective, but, ultimately, an aberration.[52]

Big money, then, elicited a range of critiques. My interviewees said Avahan created hierarchies within communities; monetized participation and dampened activism; set up a new, unsustainable parallel service delivery system; took too much credit for government and civil society successes; and focused on research and data collection at the expense of community needs. At the same time, in the years after Avahan ended, others I interviewed were nostalgic for the Avahan years, remembering a time when AIDS programs were more flexible and less demanding, when planners were open to community input, when paperwork was less likely to be backlogged or salaries delayed, and reporting requirements were actually less stringent. Regardless of their position, my interviewees largely agreed that the AIDS response within India could not be reduced to Avahan and the Gates Foundation.

Yet the Gates Foundation did play a particularly key role in representing the Indian AIDS response in the global AIDS field. Avahan was, as Alexander puts it, "one of the most well-documented public health programmes, with over three hundred peer-reviewed journal articles, scores of monographs and media features, two Harvard Business School case studies, and significant mentions in over thirty books."[53] Data management took up a substantial portion of Avahan resources—13% of Avahan's program budget went to monitoring and evaluation, compared to 3–4% of the state's budget.[54] This data collection was embedded in a "data use culture," in which everyone from program directors to grassroots peer educators was habituated to the importance of collecting, interpreting, and acting on data.[55] Avahan documents emphasized the use of quantitative data in designing programs, monitoring their progress, and evaluating their results. A "learning model"[56] meant results were always being documented and assessed, and problems recorded to inform future efforts. One article by researchers at the Gates Foundation, subtitled "How Did India Do It?" argued that India offered lessons for other countries because of its "intelligent and integrated use of data."[57] The "know your epidemic, know your response" approach used data to determine where technical and financial resources were most needed. Avahan thus played a key role in how experiences of India's AIDS response were packaged and circulated in global medical journals and institutions. Even if the Gates Foundation's role within Indian AIDS programs was contested, this academic and journalistic documentation amplified its importance.

Through this abiding focus on generating evidence, Karnataka's HIV prevention efforts are well documented. The agency coordinating Avahan programs in Karnataka, KHPT, produced training manuals, toolkits, and guidelines. I collected a stack of pamphlets and reports KHPT had produced. Academic articles quantified the work of sex worker, sexual minority, and transgender organizations. For example, an evaluation of Karnataka's program reported that it had reached 60,000 sex workers, referred 46,000 to "social entitlements" like voter ID cards and ration cards, supported violence in 4,600 incidents, and seen a 50% increase in positive media reports about sex work.[58] This documentation helped Karnataka become an example that circulated in the global AIDS field. The UNAIDS 2010 *Global Report*, for example, noted, citing Avahan-funded research,[59] that "the Indian state of Karnataka has shown evidence that intensive HIV prevention efforts among female sex workers can be highly effective."[60]

THE MAKING OF A MODEL

One of the big takeaways that Avahan emphasized from India's AIDS response was its focus on *key populations*, or *most-at-risk populations* (MARPS), revised terms for the high-risk groups that India's HIV prevention efforts centered.[61] The innovation of putting "key populations first" should be, Avahan documents said, "game-changing for the global AIDS response."[62] The insight was taken up in the global AIDS field by a range of experts and institutions. Drawing on evidence from India, the WHO promoted a focus on key populations as a neglected element of AIDS strategies in sub-Saharan Africa.[63] The World Bank offered epidemiological models that estimated the potential effects of scaling up such programs on HIV infections.[64] The impact was estimated to be greatest in countries such as Kenya, with both high HIV prevalence among sex workers and in the general population.

At a time when national AIDS budgets were increasingly strapped, targeted prevention programs for key populations held considerable appeal. Overall, the World Bank predicted that scaling up HIV prevention programs for sex workers would avert 20,683 new HIV seroconversions among adults in Kenya between 2012 and 2016[65] and save US$8.6 million in treatment costs.[66] Reducing violence against sex workers alone in Kenya could avert 5,300 new seroconversions among sex workers and 10,000 in the general population within five years.[67] These projections justified community empowerment programs in terms of cost-effectiveness and scale.

In making the case for focusing on key populations, quantification facilitated the abstraction of results from the Indian context so they could circulate transnationally. For example, the World Bank projections relied on an estimate that a sex-worker–focused response would reduce inconsistent condom use by 51%. This estimate was taken from a systematic review of ten peer-reviewed studies, most of which (seven) were from India, and nearly half of which (four) were published out of the Avahan program (three from Karnataka, and one from Andhra Pradesh).[68] But once abstracted into a number, the intricacies of these Indian contexts disappeared. When I asked George, a Kenyan AIDS official, if he had faced resistance in discussing an Indian model in Kenyan policy circles, he explained that he usually de-emphasized the Indian aspects of the model. "We're not marketing it as the Indian model," he said, "We're marketing it as a model that has worked elsewhere." The particularities of Indian programs faded from view with the model's quantification, publication in peer-reviewed journals, and dissemination through institutions like the World Bank and UNAIDS. Through the power of numbers, India's AIDS response became simply "a model that has worked."

Aside from circulating quantitative evidence in research publications, global institutions also used more direct strategies to disseminate Indian approaches to HIV prevention across Africa, including funding learning exchanges, country visits, and global conferences. For example, the Gates Foundation funded initiatives to promote India-Africa partnerships that helped shape national AIDS policies. The India Learning Network (ILN), which focused on Thailand, Bangladesh, Sri Lanka, Ghana, Ethiopia, Zambia, Uganda, Nigeria, Tanzania, and Mozambique, helped to develop the 2014–2015 National HIV/AIDS Prevention Plan in Nigeria, provided input into the *National Multisectoral Framework for HIV/AIDS in Tanzania*, and inspired a new effort to map key populations in Uganda. The ILN final report concluded that, despite some limitations, "learnings from India" were a "game changer in the African HIV program."[69]

During my fieldwork, I saw several examples of how Avahan's focus had shifted to translating its successes for global circulation, and, in particular, for adaptation in African countries. Several NGOs and CBOs I visited also had hosted visitors from sub-Saharan Africa. Ashodaya Academy in Mysore,[70] a wing of Ashodaya Samithi, provided training to sex worker organizations across the Asia-Pacific region and in sub-Saharan Africa. When I visited one organization in Bangalore, the director, in order to introduce his organization to me, showed me a PowerPoint presentation that he had given earlier that week to a visiting delegation from Kenya. Another time, I sat in on a presentation about Karnataka's HIV prevention programs for a visiting delegation from Nigeria in which the presenters explained how many peer educators to hire, how many contacts each peer educator had, and how many visits each made to the drop-in center every month. The visitors asked about the nitty-gritty of the program, including how to map a key population, track individuals, and assess results, down to the level of spreadsheets. Numbers—in the form of graphs and tables indicating the effects of HIV prevention interventions on risk behaviors, levels of violence, and HIV prevalence—played a key role in affirming the success of Indian HIV prevention in these contexts of transnational exchange.

It was not only Indian AIDS experts who shifted the focus to the quantitative aspects of HIV prevention programs. Particularly when ideas like empowerment and rights seemed untranslatable to their contexts, or working with queer organizations or sex worker collectives seemed politically unviable, strategies of enumeration became key to what African visitors could take away from the Indian experience. In a series of videos I watched on their reactions to KHPT training, for example, visitors from Tanzania, Uganda, and Nigeria answered a list of questions aloud, one by one, at a desk, with a combination of insight and bemusement. While a few mentioned the sustainability offered by working with community organizations, they hinted at the difficulties of replicating programs from a context in which "human rights are respected" and "there seems to be little stigma around sex work." On the other hand, almost all the participants mentioned the value of mapping key populations by building regular tracking and monitoring systems. A visitor from Nigeria noted, "We need to get the government to accept people in sex work. They are deeply stigmatized. There are differences in culture and context. . . . It's nice to see that sex workers here are so empowered." But her big lesson was different: "Look at your data and listen to what your data is telling you, and then align your activities with what the data is saying." She had learned that HIV prevention programs responded to data—not necessarily to politics.

FROM INDIA TO KENYA

One example of this model-making—produced and circulated through the global AIDS field—was the adaptation of Indian HIV prevention programs in Kenya. Engagements with researchers and activists from India played an important role in the Kenyan government's shift in HIV prevention in the 2010s. Kenyan AIDS agencies and supporting organizations drew on Indian experiences to conduct training, introduce new prevention programs, and help rewrite the *National Guidelines for HIV/STI Programs for Sex Workers.* These Indian experiences circulated through the research publications and statistical models that consolidated global best practices.

The core of Kenyan learning from India, my interviewees suggested, was to shift the focus of HIV prevention to key populations. The Kenyan government's efforts to reach key populations were still relatively new. Early rounds of AIDS policy made no specific effort to address these groups. Under the first Kenya National AIDS Strategic Plan (KNASP), rolled out in 2000, the government of Kenya opened HIV testing sites, conducted awareness campaigns, set up blood transfusion centers, and began providing limited antiretroviral treatment for people with AIDS. Commercial sex workers were mentioned once in the national strategic plan as a target group, along with long-distance drivers, nomads, beach communities, slum and border town residents, security forces, women and girls, and adolescents, but men who have sex with men and IV drug users were not mentioned at all. Though some of the earliest studies of HIV and sex work were done in Kenya,[71] this research had not been centrally integrated into national policy.

This relatively limited policy focus on key populations began to shift in the mid-2000s. The second five-year plan, KNASP II, included the need to target "vulnerable groups"[72] and listed a focus on prevention of new infections "in both vulnerable groups and the general population."[73] Overall, though, the plan still prioritized testing, treatment, and blood safety over interventions specifically for sex workers, sexual minorities, and transgender people. Budget allocations reflected these priorities. About 24% of the KNASP II budget for 2005–2010 was devoted to prevention programs. Of this prevention budget, 0.4% was devoted to programs for sex workers and their clients, and 2.5% to "other vulnerable groups" (including men who have sex with men and IV drug users), as opposed to 22% for youth HIV prevention programs.[74]

It was eventually research drawing on global statistical projections that pushed the Kenyan government to rethink this limited focus on preventing HIV in key populations. Starting in 2005, several research reports were released that argued for increased programmatic focus on sex workers and other MARPS. The *Behavioral Surveillance Survey* (BSS) in Kenya, conducted in 2002 but published in 2005 in collaboration with the US Centers for Disease Control and Prevention and Family Health International, defined populations "at particular risk" as youth, female sex workers, and migrant men,[75] and it argued for increased attention to the "groups driving the epidemic."[76]

The Kenya Modes of Transmission analysis, conducted between 2007 and 2008 and released in 2009, was particularly influential. The Modes of Transmission approach, first developed in 2002 by UNAIDS and the Futures Group (a development consulting firm) in Southeast Asia and piloted in Kenya,[77] was part of a UNAIDS push to streamline AIDS programs worldwide and focus resources based on epidemiological data. The Modes of Transmission analysis was piloted in Kenya, revised, and then tested again in 2008, this time in Kenya, Uganda, Mozambique, Lesotho, and Swaziland. By 2012, the model had been used in forty-four countries to identify at-risk populations.

The Kenya Modes of Transmission analysis argued much more forcefully than the BSS for renewed attention to sex workers and men who have sex with men. The report argued that Kenya had a mixed epidemic, one that included both high general prevalence and even higher prevalence among key populations, and that existing KNASP strategies "do not fit with the epidemiological evidence."[78] Programs should instead expand their focus on prevention, specifically among sex workers, their clients, men who have sex with men, and prisoners, groups who together accounted for, according to the analysis, 29.3% of new HIV infections nationwide.[79] The analysis found that heterosexual sex within a union or "regular partnership" (44.1%) and "casual heterosexual sex" (20.3%) still accounted for the majority of infections, but the report's policy recommendations mainly focused on the other risk groups.[80] Overall, the report pushed for "full scale-up of prevention strategies,"[81] which were currently fragmented and implemented through a range of NGOs and faith-based organizations without systematic coordination.

Anthropologist Manjari Mahajan writes about what she calls global foreknowledge—the use of existing assumptions to predetermine what kind of quantitative evidence is collected, ultimately confirming existing assumptions in a kind of self-fulfilling prophecy.[82] Those involved in the Modes of Transmission analysis acknowledged the limitations of global foreknowledge. The categories used in the Modes of Transmission analysis predetermined the potential outcomes: if data existed for a category of women called female sex workers and this category was then included in epidemiological models, the model would then confirm that this group contributed significantly to the AIDS epidemic at large. The results of analysis were thus, in a way, known from the start. One researcher I interviewed concurred: "If you don't look for it, you're not going to find it." The Modes of Transmission model was also not open to the addition of new categories.[83] He explained, "All sorts of populations can be considered to be at high risk of AIDS—you know, babies, teenage girls, out-of-work youth, truck drivers. It's a long list. And UNAIDS at that time had just sort of coined the term MARPS. And to their definition, MARPS were sex workers, IDUs, MSM. That was the category that we were supposed to populate. And so any other groups were added grudgingly." From this researcher's perspective, modeling was an exercise riddled with uncertainty, whose wide application seemed unwarranted:

> The secret of the problems with modeling is that a lot of these global reports that you see on, you know, the incidence of tonsillitis in Ghana is based on very, very limited data. People have found a paper or two with a sample group of a few dozen, and extrapolated that into the whole country. So, I wouldn't say that the Kenya Modes of Transmission study was that extreme, but I must also confess that sitting in meetings over the last few years, and seeing our study being so widely quoted, and seeing

policy being based on it, also recognizing that some of those conclusions were not the strongest conclusions we could have had, makes me a little bit uncomfortable.

These observations pointed to the limits of quantitative exercises. Researchers themselves recognized that the numbers they produced only partially reflected social realities and solidified predetermined categories of risk. Despite these reservations, the study was taken up for policy development. The study's estimate that a third of infections were concentrated in key populations often came up in my interviews. The Kenya AIDS Indicator Survey (KAIS), released at the same time, identified geographic regions and other demographic patterns in HIV prevalence.[84] Together, the two studies inspired the National AIDS Control Council (NACC) to reformulate its national strategy two years early. A foreword by the minister of state for special programs cited the two studies and noted that the policy focused on the prevention of new infections as well as care and support of people living with HIV.[85] The policy had a "crosscutting focus" on "most-at-risk and vulnerable populations (MARPs),"[86] with sex workers, drug users, and men who have sex with men the "primary MARPs."[87]

Through the magic of quantification, the Modes of Transmission analysis and the KAIS, though largely using existing data and then analyzing them against assumptions generated by UNAIDS, became evidence of Kenyan trends. "It's basically based on the evidence," said a Kenyan program officer, when I asked how Kenya's National AIDS and STI Control Programme (NASCOP) had determined the most important key populations. Harry, a NASCOP official, said the studies had made a difference when political pressure had not: "There has been, of course, pressure among key populations, before even [the] Modes of Transmission study and the KAIS. But it's after that evidence was generated that they thought there would be a national coordination and leadership by NASCOP. So . . . it's just responding to the evidence, because previously we did not have hard evidence as regarding to what key populations are contributing to." The categories generated by the Modes of Transmission analysis, which were defined according to UNAIDS standards, became standard categories in the Kenyan policy, with alternative categories, such as prisoners or the military, now regional variations to be evaluated on a case-by-case basis. When I asked if there were other relevant categories, Harry explained, "Everyone will come and tell you in my area these are the key populations. So [the policy] should avoid that, to use focus."

A new policy focus on key populations did not reflect a shift in budget. In KNASP III, sex worker programs officially comprised 0.7% of the budget,[88] an increase from 0.1% in the previous policy. Targeted prevention programs were relatively inexpensive compared to treatment at a large scale. George explained, "We were investing where we were not getting much in terms of prevention. So . . . with the review of the KNASP . . . there was a lot of focus on designing programs that would then target these key populations because we needed to close the tap where the greatest infections were coming from." Targeting key populations was thus a better investment: it would lower costs by controlling the epidemic at its source.

THE SIMPLE THINGS IN LIFE

On paper, KNASP III widened the range of concerns to be included in HIV prevention programs with key populations to include social, political, and economic aspects of their lives. The policy discussed issues such as the "criminalization of MARPs' high-risk behavior" because of "religious and cultural resistance," their marginalization from public sector services, and "denial and social intolerance."[89] Interventions would address "root causes of vulnerability" including "beliefs and values around masculinity and femininity."[90] The authors called for a "rights-based approach" where "civil society will be strongly involved."[91] The accompanying *National Guidelines for HIV/STI Programs for Sex Workers* suggested following participatory processes that empowered sex workers and built consensus.[92] "Community mobilization" programs would "encourage these individuals to organize themselves and advocate for their health and human rights.[93]

Despite this broad mandate, some interviewees told me that Kenyan HIV prevention programs with key populations would begin with a narrower focus on condom distribution, HIV testing, and monitoring and move into community mobilization later. They drew inspiration from the Indian model of focusing on key populations, but they focused on the quantitative aspects of the model, such as planning and data management. In the words of one AIDS expert who had moved from India to Kenya, "the simple things in life," such as condom distribution and monitoring, must precede concerns about advocacy or structural change:

I know people want to hear things like community mobilization, advocacy, and violence, and this and that. They can come later. You see,
I can't talk about advocacy if I'm working with ten sex workers. . . .
when the estimates are in the thousands. So my point is that first you
reach the thousand. Do some programming with them. . . . Then you
can talk about other things. . . . The point is that keep it simple in
the beginning. The simple things in life. How many are there? How
many have you reached? How many are coming to clinics? How many
condoms are going? Is it enough? Things like that. Then you can talk
about crisis, violence, this, that, mobilization, group building, so on
and so forth.

For this interviewee, mobilization "sounds very nice, goody-goody job, a
bit more soft-core in nature," and the priority was "hardcore prevention"
before getting into the "frills of the program." In the context of this approach focused on the "simple things in life," community mobilization
took on a different meaning than it had in India. In India, it focused on
empowerment programs, community-building, and even activism. But in
Kenya, program staff I interviewed described it as "mobilizing sex workers
for information and services," with efficient and targeted outreach, and
individualized tracking and assessment. In Kenya's guidelines for working with key populations, the "enabling environment" for HIV prevention
was defined as "access to appropriate, affordable, acceptable and accessible
health services without being penalized."[94] Indian guidelines defined it as
an environment "wherein those infected and affected by HIV could lead a
life of dignity free from stigma and discrimination."[95] As the Indian model
traveled, it narrowed in scope.

As dissemination proceeded, the quantitative aspects of the Indian model
continued to predominate. Starting in 2012, Kenya's NASCOP began to form
model programs that could serve as a training ground for organizations
working with sex workers, sexual minorities, and transgender people for
HIV prevention, inspired in part by Indian HIV prevention programs. It
partnered with organizations in Mombasa—the International Centre for
Reproductive Health–Kenya[96]—and in Nairobi—the Sex Workers' Outreach
Project (SWOP),[97] with support from the Bar Hostesses' Empowerment and
Support Program[98] and the Kenya Sex Workers' Alliance[99]—to facilitate these
Learning Sites.

I heard a range of perspectives on the goals of the Learning Sites and what they had taken from India, but most focused on data. One researcher in Mombasa saw the benefit of the Indian model as largely related to an intensification of individualized surveillance: "We have been trying and asking ourselves questions. . . . how many sex workers are we reaching in our program? But we never had a clear, straightforward answer. Because in . . . previous peer education sessions, sex workers will hold those sessions with a mixture of some other women who are within that locality. Therefore you will not exactly know who is a sex worker and who is not. Although you can know, but you will not know exactly how many. Because we were not keeping records of individual names." For him, tools from India allowed for individualized tracking. I heard about the value of this kind of micro-planning over and over in my interviews. Another program officer in Mombasa noted that "one of the key things that I've said I've learned from the Indian model that was very, very good was the micro-planning. I think that's the one key thing that I would take from that. That we had not thought about it in that way. You micro-plan for each and every individual."

These micro-planning efforts, with their high targets, heavy paperwork, and low pay, exhausted peer educators, who echoed what I often heard from peer educators in India. One peer educator, Anne, noted, "Something I really, really don't like about the organization is about the recruitment. . . . we have to recruit over sixty people, that's a lot . . . we are several there, and all of us have to bring over these people, it's a very big challenge. . . . and we have a lot of paperwork! It's too tiresome! . . . [for] three thousand [KSh, or about US$27] . . . That is too, too little." These targets and documentation strategies were an important part of what had traveled to Anne's organization from Indian models. When I introduced myself to a nurse at a sex worker clinic in Mombasa, she told me that they were "trying to copy India here in this office." "We used to give a box of condoms to everyone," she said, "but now we have to ask them: how many sex acts do you do? How many partners?" Copying India, for this nurse, looked very different from the sexual politics that this book has documented. It meant collecting and using numbers, even when it brought an awkward rigidity to the relationships the clinic had already built.

NUMBERS AND SEXUAL POLITICS

Questions about whether the Indian model actually could be translated to the Kenyan context often came up in my interviews. In everyday conversation, those involved in adapting the Indian model, both in India and in Kenya, knew they had been asked to package a program that had taken years of conflict and struggle to build. They knew they were exporting it to new contexts with far less time and resources than they needed. As they navigated the complexity of the exchange, they focused on the basics—biomedical intervention now focused on key populations, with an emphasis on monitoring and tracking—while the activist engagements that had shaped the Indian model fell by the wayside. As this chapter has shown, numbers and documentation played a role at every stage. In India, participatory programs with sex workers, sexual minorities, and transgender people were documented and reports and academic articles published. In Kenya, international standards and statistical projections were adapted and new programs initiated.

The version of the Indian AIDS response that policymakers attempted to replicate in Kenya was distinct from what it had been in India. The sources of success in India had emerged in the cracks in coercive public health programs, in collective mobilizations that had pushed back against state and donor excesses, and in critiques that had been absorbed, renegotiated, and pushed once more. Communities could not just be mobilized by technocrats, nor could sex workers, sexual minorities, and transgender people become engaged in the process through epidemiological modeling. Through the process of quantification, the Indian AIDS response was ultimately stripped down from its political complexities into a series of epidemiological strategies, surveillance mechanisms, and management tricks—"the simple things in life."

Quantification enabled an abstraction of AIDS programs from their political and social contexts. But in practice, exchanges between Indian and Kenyan HIV prevention programs resisted this abstraction. For both Indian and Kenyan AIDS officials, the process of translating Indian experiences into the Kenyan context uncovered fundamental assumptions about what it meant to be Indian and Kenyan, and gave both the opportunity to define and reformulate their understandings of each country's place in the global AIDS field. The next chapter turns to the meanings that accompanied the travel of AIDS programs for key populations from India to Kenya. As each country jostled for attention on the world stage, AIDS success became more than just an abstraction of complex local experience into a replicable model. It tapped into deeper questions about each country's place in the global order.

7 | INDIA IN AFRICA

A FEW WEEKS AFTER ARRIVING in Nairobi, I attended a talk by a prominent North American public health researcher about AIDS programs in Karnataka. The audience members were all AIDS researchers and program planners who supported the Kenyan government's HIV prevention programs, in part by drawing on Indian experiences of HIV prevention. The speaker, personable and precise, described peer education projects with sex workers, sexual minorities, and transgender people in India and analyzed their results. At the end of the talk, he asked the Indian staff about their experiences working in Kenya. "It's so pleasant to work here," said one. "There's a real civility and politeness. Not like India!"

In recent years, *South-South partnership* has gained currency as a buzzword[1] in international development circles.[2] The talk fit the buzz: researchers were sharing an HIV prevention model that could be translated from one global South context to another. What had worked in India had the potential to work in Kenya, too. The speaker's graphs and charts rendered the complicated sexual politics of AIDS in India and Kenya legible and manageable. His presentation reinforced the Indian program's reproducibility: it was clear, well-documented, and accessible, and these features made it easier to emulate. But the Indian staff member's response hints at something more than the circulation of a technical fix. It highlights the symbolic stakes of this

South-South relationship. She was using her experience in Kenya to develop an insight into what India was like, marking a contrast, a limit against which she defined what it meant to be Indian. Working across India and Kenya pushed researchers to reexamine the differences between India and Kenya, especially in relation to political and sexual life.

Once AIDS experts translated complex political struggles into models of HIV prevention that could be circulated in the global AIDS field in the form of easily digestible numbers, they were put to use. This chapter turns to the implementation of, and debates over, traveling best practices as they moved across uneven postcolonial geographies.[3] South-South collaborations were not simply exchanges of technical tools or a diffusion of innovations.[4] Instead, this chapter argues that, despite the quantification of the Indian AIDS response, questions about the similarities and differences between India and Kenya informed how a range of AIDS experts approached the exchange. In the global AIDS field, India's AIDS successes were defined in contrast to Kenya's less advanced state capacity. In the process, the Indian state was reimagined: once overstretched, uneven, and corrupt, it was now capable, omniscient, and technically advanced. Once a conservative state unwilling to confront an imminent crisis that would follow the trajectory of AIDS in Africa, India was now a model of HIV prevention. India was the "technological *above* to an underdeveloped *below*."[5] But in the everyday process of South-South exchange, program officers often encountered the differences between India and Kenya as more complex than global institutions might suggest. They came up against the many ways in which Indian HIV prevention programs could not be so easily translated.

When global experts spoke of India's effective AIDS response in relation to Kenya's inability to manage its epidemic, they did not do so in a historical vacuum. Rather, they built on colonial hierarchies that were fundamentally racialized and sexualized. Experts mobilized ideas of the Indian state as more technically skilled and of its population as more sexually restrained than a more administratively dependent and sexually promiscuous Africa. These tropes also evoked Cold War imaginaries of Indian-African solidarity and bold images of India's post-liberalization entry onto the world stage as a major economic power.[6]

Efforts at South-South collaboration reveal how these deep-seated ideas about race, gender, sexuality, and national difference shape relations in the global AIDS field.[7] Global institutions like the Gates Foundation, the WHO, and UNAIDS and the quantitative measures they created assessed nation-states as successes and failures in responding to the AIDS crisis. North American and European experts set the terms of South-South comparisons, like the North American researcher at the talk in Nairobi. In my interviews, Indian experts often remarked with pride that the Indian AIDS response had received global acclaim and was considered a model for the AIDS response. Yet, in the practice of exchanging notes on HIV prevention, they acknowledged that replicating the model, and taking Indian HIV prevention outside of the political context in which it had been developed, was more difficult than it seemed.

IMAGINING INDIA IN AFRICA

When scholars analyze the travel of best practices and South-South partnerships, they often locate it in dynamics of globalization and neoliberalization in the 1990s and 2000s.[8] But understanding the symbolic stakes of India-Kenya exchange requires examining a longer historical lineage, as well as attention to how gendered and sexual dynamics undergird transnational administrative exchanges. For example, the circulation of governance techniques from India to Africa occurred regularly in the British Empire, from the use of fingerprinting techniques[9] to the regulation of prostitution and homosexuality[10] in the nineteenth century. Colonial officials tested techniques of statecraft in India before implementing them in Africa. As feminist historian Antoinette Burton has shown, they saw Indian civilization as more advanced within a global racialized hierarchy, higher than Africa but lower than Europe. Discourses of gender and sexuality anchored such civilizational orders.[11] Indian nationalists, most famously Gandhi, formed their own self-image in relation to Africans. Scholars have shown how both Indian immigrants in Africa[12] and Indian nationalists within India[13] constructed Africa as primitive in contrast to India's advancement. Indian freedom fighters wrote of East Africa as "India's America" or a "second India,"[14] which marked the racial limits of Indianness.

After India's independence, Indian discourses about Africa retained much of the colonial hierarchy of nations, revealing the underlying idea that, as

Burton puts it, "Africa's future will be made by drawing on history that India has already passed through, developed out of, and can now export as a kind of technopolitical good to desperate black colonial subjects whose destiny is apparently to approximate the political, economic, and social forms of their Indian betters."[15] Afro-Asian solidarity conferences in the 1950s and 1960s, in Bandung, Belgrade, Cairo, Conakry, and Moshi, celebrated the possibilities of African-Asian connections but retained this hierarchical relation.[16] India's first prime minister, Jawaharlal Nehru, in the midst of the Cold War, envisioned a utopian African-Asian solidarity that positioned Africa as "the junior African 'other.'"[17] In 1947, Nehru noted, "We of Asia have a special responsibility to the peoples of Africa. We must help them to their rightful place in the human family."[18]

Since the 1990s, India[19] has followed China in becoming an investor in African countries.[20] Several major Indian companies, both state-owned and private, have invested in Africa's oil, natural gas, and manufacturing industries. These relationships extend to humanitarian assistance and development funding; for example, India has pledged US$1 million toward sustainable development and poverty alleviation in Africa, is the largest contributor of UN peacekeepers in Africa, and has also provided smaller-scale humanitarian assistance. India has provided more than $1 billion in technical assistance and training to personnel in African development programs.[21] Indian drugs have become crucial to AIDS treatment in Africa.[22] India's prime minister Narendra Modi aims to expand bilateral trade with the continent to $150 billion by 2023, as part of a 2017 vision for an Asia-Africa Growth Corridor that focuses on agriculture, health care, and pharmaceuticals.[23] Though the AIDS partnerships in this chapter were funded by global donors, not the Indian government, they must be understood within this geopolitical context, as India charts a path to economic and geopolitical influence in "the new scramble for Africa."[24] For both Indian and Kenyan AIDS experts, South-South exchanges became sites for reproducing and sometimes challenging discourses about the global order and where they fit within it.

HIV EXCEPTIONALISM IN KENYA AND INDIA

One way to understand the positions of India and Kenya in the global AIDS field is to consider their epidemiological trajectories and responses. By the mid-2000s in India, the crisis was predicted; in Kenya, it had already arrived.

For example, in 2011, both countries had decreasing estimated adult HIV prevalence, but Kenya's was much higher, having decreased from 8.5% to 6.2% between 2001 and 2011,[25] compared to India's prevalence having decreased from 0.4% to 0.3% between 2001 and 2009.[26] Among female sex workers, a widely cited *Lancet* meta-analysis estimated an HIV prevalence of 13.7% in India and 45.1% in Kenya.[27] Despite the urgency of the crisis, the Kenyan state responded to the AIDS epidemic relatively late: President Moi declared the epidemic a national emergency only in 2000. By then, international organizations had already stepped in, helping create conditions in which donors, NGOs, and state agencies operated in isolation and sometimes competition. Thus, in contrast to the Indian state, the Kenyan AIDS response was more dependent on donor funding. It played a more circumscribed role in coordinating AIDS programs, and donor agendas were more likely to overwhelm national agendas or engagements with social movements.

In line with the HIV exceptionalism[28] scholars have documented, Kenyan AIDS programs in the 2000s received disproportionate international funding in comparison to other health sectors in Kenya. Kenya had a relatively higher budget than India's for AIDS: in 2009, Kenya's AIDS budget was $687.3 million,[29] compared to India's $140 million.[30] One way to index HIV exceptionalism is to compare foreign funding for AIDS and the health sector. As Figures 1 and 2 show,[31] Kenya saw official development funding commitments for AIDS outstrip funding for the health sector after 2002, while in India, this only happened in 2007.

Overall, Kenya's AIDS budget was composed of funding from fewer sources, mainly USAID, than India's AIDS budget.[32] Under its third strategic plan, the Kenyan government reported that it contributed only 6% of its AIDS budget for 2009/10 to 2012/13,[33] while the Indian government reported contributing 40.8% of the Indian AIDS budget for 2007 to 2012.[34] Kenya's reliance on US funding is particularly significant because of the US government's restriction on funding agencies that do not have an explicit policy opposing prostitution,[35] agencies which are often more activist- or rights-based organizations. US bilateral aid comprised, on average, 83% of official development assistance for STD and AIDS control in Kenya and 24% in India between 2005 and 2015.[36] According to the National AIDS Control Council, of Kenya's AIDS budget in 2009/10, 81% came from the US government under the President's Emergency Plan for AIDS Relief (PEPFAR),[37] USAID, and

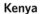

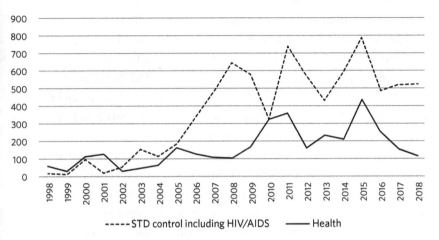

FIGURE 1. Official development assistance to Kenya for STD control, including HIV, exceeded funding for the health sector from 2002 to 2018. Data for 1998 to 2018 is displayed in millions of constant 2018 US dollars. Source: OECD Creditor Reporting System.

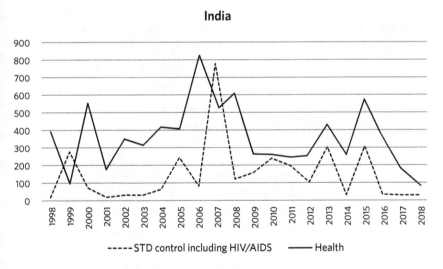

FIGURE 2. Official development assistance to India for STD control, including HIV, only exceeded funding for the health sector in 2007. Data for 1998 to 2018 is displayed in millions of constant 2018 US dollars. Source: OECD Creditor Reporting System.

the Centers for Disease Control and Prevention.[38] In comparison to Kenya's, India's budget was relatively less reliant on bilateral donors and especially on US government funding. Unlike Kenya, India was not a PEPFAR focus country, and its bilateral donors included a wider variety of countries, including Australia, the UK, Canada, and the Netherlands. The largest multilateral sources of funding for Indian AIDS programs were the World Bank, the Global Fund, the UK's Department for International Development, and the Gates Foundation.[39] As a result, US prostitution policy had relatively limited influence on its HIV prevention programs.

The larger role of donors in the Kenyan AIDS response meant local organizations had to respond to multiple demands from different donors. Often, several donors operated in one place. Interviewees at all the organizations I visited mentioned competition for funds between those working in the same area as a key challenge, in addition to the multiple program priorities donors imposed. This competition also incentivized NGOs to conduct outreach in more accessible places to improve outcome numbers, leading to uneven coverage. One HIV expert noted:

> NGOs are more accountable to the donors than to the government. Donors have increasingly tightened their strings so they are expecting more for less . . . so the space is crowded, so everybody is fighting for space. . . . In some places they have up to six implementing partners reaching out to the same female sex workers within the same location. . . . Some of them, three or four of them are from the same funding agency . . . The low hanging fruits are those places, people that you can easily reach. . . . So everybody comes to the same club that is in town.

Faced with this pressure, Kenyan NGO staff discussed the limitations of donor culture much more frequently than my Indian interviewees did. In India, NGO leaders explained, donors might have priorities but they were rarely successful in imposing their agendas on organizations entirely, even the powerful Gates Foundation. In Kenya, selling one's contribution to donors was a prerequisite to any work, and if an organization lost its funding, another group would be there to take its place. In this context, sex worker, sexual minority, and transgender organizations in Kenya felt highly circumscribed when they made demands on or imposed conditions on state and donor involvement. They could not refuse funding, as SANGRAM in India famously did.[40] And if they objected to how the AIDS response was unfolding, rather than protesting or pressuring a single state-affiliated coordinating agency, they had a complex array of faraway donors to tackle.

THE POLITICS OF COMPARISON

In addition to these epidemiological and institutional differences, my interviewees also observed and debated political and social differences between the AIDS responses in India and Kenya. One Indian staff member focused on culture: she said Kenyans were less disruptive, more accepting of donor authority than Indians were. There was no culture of "shouting and screaming" or protesting in Kenya, like in India. In a traffic jam in Nairobi, she said, people would sit patiently for hours. In Bangalore they would have spent so much time getting out of their cars, picking fights, and honking their horns that they would have started a new traffic jam. There was, she said, less of a "spirit of voluntarism" among sex workers in Kenya. Kenyans I interviewed, too, articulated differences between Kenyan and Indian political cultures, saying Kenyans were conservative and Indians were tolerant and outgoing. Mercy, a sex worker activist who had visited India through an exchange program funded by an AIDS donor, reflected,

> You know . . . in India, the community is close and together with that togetherness. In Kenya we don't have that togetherness. So for them implementing projects is very easy. They can bring sex workers together, bring kids of sex workers together to go to school, they can even say sex workers should go to this brothel. But in Kenya it's hard. [Why?] Because of the culture I guess. The way we are brought up. Even where I stay in my apartment, I don't know my neighbor. I don't even know my neighbor, and it's not by default but it's the way I'm raised up. I don't care about my friend or who's around me. . . . But I realized in India, eating, you have to eat together. Sitting, you sit together. In Kenya, no no no no.

I was surprised to hear Mercy make this comparison. When I had met her, we had sat together with others from her organization and laughed over lunch. Mercy herself seemed to have close relationships with sex workers at her organization. She had tracked down a sex worker organization after losing her mother and struggling with her siblings to pay the bills, and she had used her salary there to pay her way through college. She described herself—and others agreed with her—as an organizational success story. Nevertheless, she aligned with Indian colleagues in describing Kenyan culture as less supportive than India's. Her account aligned with other binary characterizations other interviewees presented: Kenya's political culture was more pliable and conservative, India more progressive and independent.

These assessments of political culture entailed a parallel analysis of the state. According to my interviewees, the Kenyan state was less autonomous than the Indian state and depended more on global donor control. As one Indian AIDS expert working in Kenya put it,

> The other difference is that, [if] you take the Indian government and Kenya, once the government of India spends the money, if they control the money, they control all the decisions around it as well. You get the point? . . . Government of India would say, well, this is our national mandate, these are the national guidelines, this is our gap, so why don't you go over there and fill up the gap. . . . In Kenya it's the reverse. . . . If you ask [the government] today how much money comes in for the HIV program, they don't have an answer. Because they don't know. . . . The government is not in control or in charge of funding and programming.

To Indian experts, the role of global donors in Kenya's AIDS response left Kenyan state officials unable to assert priorities or coordinate efforts. He went on to attribute the difference to Kenyan political culture. "People don't want to be assertive. This is a very polite country, you see. We [Indians] are not so polite. That's the problem. People over here are very polite so they don't stand their ground, don't ask for things." The language of Indian innovation and Kenya's desire to catch up surfaced often in my conversations with AIDS experts. Regarding donor coordination, one interviewee noted, "India was like that in 2006. . . . in Kenya they're still in 2004. I'm sure it'll improve." Another HIV expert based in India explained, "Indian economy after eighties changed. The government takes a lot of shots, even with donors. They say we don't want your money; if you want you give according to our conditions. But there [in Africa] it is still—they are like old India. Their economy is not strong, so the donor dictates the terms." Here, India was a few years "ahead" of Kenya, and Kenya would eventually "improve" to look more like India, more independent in relation to Europe and North America. These accounts made clear a temporal hierarchy of autonomy from donors.

My interviewees also compared Indian and Kenyan sexual cultures. While both Indian and Kenyan interviewees saw Kenya as more conservative than India, often linking this conservatism to Christian and Muslim clergy, they nevertheless positioned Kenyan sex workers as more sexually open and less hidden than their Indian counterparts. As one interviewee put it, "In India you'd need a torch [flashlight] to find a sex worker, you know. It's such a pain. In Kenya you don't have to do that actually. Walk into any bar, you find sex workers. Walk into any street, you find sex workers." He emphasized Kenyan sex workers' ubiquity and visibility, as opposed to Indian sex workers, who more easily blended into the crowd.

More grassroots HIV prevention workers, including sex workers, also drew this contrast between visible and sexually open Kenyan sex workers and more carefully hidden, discreet Indian sex workers, and between more stigmatized Kenyan gay men and more accepted Indian gay men. One sex worker in Mombasa I interviewed worked as a peer supervisor and had been part of HIV prevention programs for several years. She also worked as a hairdresser. When I met her she was dressed in a fabulous purple leopard print with matching eyeshadow. She said she loved to dress up, to not look like a "poor person." "Sex work in India is safe," she said. "People don't know who is a sex worker because they wear saris and dress nicely." Kenyan sex workers, she suggested, by contrast, had to put themselves at risk by dressing the part. This difference meant sex workers faced more danger in their everyday lives. I often heard in my interviews in Kenya that sex work in India was legal, unlike in Kenya. In reality, Indian and Kenyan sex workers face similar legal restrictions,[41] but the misperception suggested that India was more tolerant of sex work and that sex workers there were more respectable (and respected).[42] Ann, an NGO director, noted, "I understand in India, there's a caste for sex work. In Kenya today, sex work is still very low, still being considered lazy and loose morals to be doing that thing, and there are always options, you're told, so many things you can do instead of selling yourself, there's always many things you can do according to the society." This analysis also appeared in an interview in Bangalore with Nikhil, an NGO staff member, who recalled a visit to South Africa. He explained that they thought their sex worker empowerment programs could not be replicated in other countries and continued,

In South Africa if you take [our NGO's] model, most sex workers will say they're looking for a husband. I'm not doing sex work. They'll be offended like hell. But they'll negotiate price with you happily. They'll negotiate price with you. But they'll say I'm not talking about sex work. Very different. Girls are early initiated into sex, and [they have] much less inhibition about approaching a man and talking about sex. Men have no inhibition at all. We were sitting in Johannesburg and we were like wow, my God, I mean, the scenario. I was holding my head and sitting, I said I can't take this. They picked up a bunch of six girls, and two or three of these men, and they stopped by and said, would you also join, we don't have enough men, so why don't you jump into the car! We're like no, we're having tea. Look at the girls! And one of them was pulling down somebody's shorts and we were like oh my God, can't even finish our tea in peace! . . . Girls are different, women are different, issues are different.

Ann and Nikhil's accounts converged in suggesting that India had a sexual culture distinct from that of African countries, but they diverged on how. Nikhil argued that sex work was more open in South Africa, that women in sex work there were less inhibited. Nikhil saw fundamental differences between South African sex workers and Indian sex workers. To him, South African sex workers were more sexually open than Indian sex workers, in a way that left him uncomfortable. While my interviews across India and Kenya did not corroborate this difference,[43] Nikhil's account of "girls" "pulling down somebody's shorts" and interrupting his tea evoked a distinct archetype of aggressive African feminine sexuality.[44] Ann, meanwhile, drew on her own archetype about Indian feminine sexuality—she linked sex work to traditional native practice, rooting it in the caste system. Each drew on these archetypes to characterize their own context as more sexually restrained than the other.

Another comparison between Africa and India that emerged in my fieldwork was a contrast between tolerance and modernity, epitomized in Indian acceptance of diverse sexualities, and the stigma and silencing of sexual minorities in Africa. This narrative, for example, emerged when African visitors interacted with Indian HIV peer educators on their study visits to India. Several of my interviewees had met groups from Kenya, Tanzania, Nigeria, and Uganda who had visited their drop-in centers. Gitesh, an outreach worker in Bangalore who identified as a double-decker, recalled a visit to his

CBO drop-in center from some Kenyan officials. They had spoken through a translator, Gitesh said, and the visitors had even taken photos. "They said if we opened up as much as you have here, where we live, they'd even shoot us. [What did you feel then?] I felt kind of happy. In our India, it's so much better, isn't it? Look, they have so many hopes, but they can't show it outside. It has to be so difficult."

For those involved in HIV prevention, the character of the AIDS epidemic and the success or failure of interventions to address it hinged on fundamental questions about Indian and Kenyan sexual politics. For Gitesh, encountering Kenyan visitors had helped him see India as a place of sexual tolerance and empathize with Kenyan sexual minorities in a new way. It allowed him to position his own experiences within a global framework, to recognize that, as he put it, "homosexuality exists there too," while taking pride in Indian tolerance.

SUBVERTING REPLICABILITY

Rather than an abstracted model that could travel from one place to another, or from one more technically advanced country to a less technically advanced one, these accounts suggested a complex set of political and sexual differences between India and Kenya that made Indian AIDS programs difficult to replicate. While some Kenyan AIDS experts were eager to take inspiration from Indian programs, others were less willing to accept the terms of transnational engagement and contested the relevance of Indian expertise. By emphasizing the differences between India and Kenya, critics in both countries challenged the logic of the traveling "good project" or best practice.

For some interviewees in Kenya, the utility of Indian HIV prevention models was obvious. When I asked if they had learned from any other countries within Africa, they usually said no. One experienced public health researcher explained,

> In terms of other countries, we will have to adopt the Indian model because it has shown to provide good results, it has shown to make a bigger impact, and it has also shown that it is more effective and efficient in delivering quality services to the sex workers. So in the African scenario, Kenya is leading in provision of services to sex workers. It has better government policies than any other country, apart from I think Senegal where sex work is legalized. So we are better off and we are more better

in relation to sex workers in African region . . . And that's why we went to borrow from India because we thought the Indian model looks more efficient, it is more evidence based, so it is good for decision making and planning. So that's why we've copied that model up to now. We've not been convinced by any other model apart from the Indian model.

This interviewee articulated a hierarchical set of relations in which India was technically advanced in comparison to Kenya, but Kenya was so technically advanced in comparison to every other African country that only India could provide a model for innovation.

The need to learn from India was not necessarily a response to the evidence. Many ostensibly Indian strategies for HIV prevention had actually been pioneered in Kenya long before they had been attempted on a large scale in India. And Kenyan sex workers indicated high levels of knowledge about HIV prevention on surveys before the government decided to focus prevention programs on them. Out of all groups covered in the Behavioral Surveillance Survey, for example, female sex workers had the highest levels of knowledge about AIDS: 60% had "no misconceptions" about the disease's transmission, and 88% had used a condom during their last sexual encounter.[45] Sex workers had been engaged in HIV prevention programs in Kenya since the start of the epidemic. However, policy documents very rarely acknowledged Kenya's existing strengths in HIV prevention. Few of my interviewees in government could identify any approaches that had been previously used in Kenya that inspired their HIV prevention activities.

On the other hand, however, some Kenyan leaders were more skeptical of Indian expertise. One interviewee exemplified this opposition to adopting Indian models:

One shoe does not fit everybody. India had their experience, but we have to be culturally sensitive. . . . We have not reached a place yet to embrace [sex work]. . . . Sometimes if you want something so much, you show people so much, we are sex workers, we're here, see us, see us, it won't work. . . . Sex workers are still very hidden. Severely hidden in Kenya. So I agree we learned so much from India, but I want us to not cut and paste. It's good we implement, but we implement what works for us. . . . So what I'm saying is that we learned so much from India. . . . but I'd like to see what is working for Kenya.

This account mobilized several arguments for the irrelevance of Indian expertise to Kenya. It was not culturally sensitive, and it was practically inefficient because sex work was hidden in Kenya. She acknowledged the hierarchical structure of the global AIDS field: Kenya had "not reached a place yet" to implement Indian-style HIV prevention. However, her conclusion diverged from the argument that adapting Indian models was fitting for Kenya's level of advancement. She argued instead that, because of its different characteristics, Kenya must forge its own path.

Skepticism of the relevance of Indian models in Kenya was not uncommon. Observers from outside Kenya noted the differences between contexts too. One interviewee explained:

> India is open to political collectivization. There is not that same process in Africa at all. They have another approach to how to manage political struggle, how to manage community empowerment. Avahan in India transported what they thought would work, but what we're finding is fracturing. Every time a group starts to get going, within two years they are collapsing. They're splintering. Unless there's an Africa consciousness to the programs—a connection to all the sex workers in Africa—until they get to that point, it will continue to erupt and fracture.

In India, too, many of the staff I interviewed were skeptical of the possibility of circulating the Indian model transnationally. "I'm not doing a ready-made model that will work in Uganda," said one program official in Karnataka. "You can distribute condoms in a day, but you can't change the whole thinking in a day." Even those centrally involved in South-South partnerships were open in discussing the limits on translating experience across countries. These accounts suggested that the Indian experience could not simply be abstracted and reapplied in a new context through quantitative modeling. It had to contend with the particular sexual politics of each place.

REINVENTING THE MODEL

The Indian HIV prevention model that circulated through the global AIDS field required state agencies to work with sex worker, sexual minority, and transgender organizations. These partnerships, as they had in India, opened space for a range of articulations. Some organizations focused more on a biomedical understanding of HIV prevention, and some oriented themselves toward social support systems, advocacy, or building political consciousness. Each type of organization took distinct lessons from Indian HIV prevention programs.

The first category of organizations saw their role centrally as health providers. When I asked a staff member at one such HIV prevention organization about her dreams for her organization, she said simply, "To account for each and every sex worker and her risk profile." It was a dream adapted to a constrained reality. Legal issues, as another interviewee put it, were "something we can't do anything about." Another said, when I asked about human rights work, "No, we are more under the public health. . . . I don't think we are crossing the boundary to go to rights." While her organization might provide a platform and rooms in which people could meet, it "stays away from that. That's not our core business. . . . internally we will not be seen carrying placards and saying we are in sex work."

These organizations generally argued that their approach was an adaptation to their context. Leaders I interviewed felt that taking on a more political or legal approach to HIV prevention, especially advocating for decriminalizing sex work and homosexuality, might endanger the AIDS response and attract violence and repression by challenging Kenyan sexual norms. A program officer explained that it was important to insist over and over to potential critics within the government that their programs were primarily focused on HIV prevention and that they were "not trying to legalize anything." In Mombasa, one of the drop-in centers for men in sex work had been set on fire. An interviewee who worked at an NGO there said emphasizing connections to the Ministry of Health, and downplaying the leadership of sex workers, sexual minorities, and transgender people, provided a measure of protection from such attacks. When they spoke about Indian HIV prevention programs, they mainly said they had learned from their Indian counterparts how to monitor more efficiently, or how to manage data better.

Not all Kenyan organizations involved in government HIV prevention programs avoided activism, though. A second category of organizations saw the Kenyan government's new interest in key populations as an opportunity to find seats at the table for activism. Their attempts to participate were not always welcomed by their more biomedically-oriented counterparts. One activist noted, "I'll say that it has been a bit challenging, because the organizations that were chosen to work with us are not sex-worker–led organizations, so when we put our ideas [forward] they think that we are so stupid, we didn't go to school, so we can't tell them anything. They feel like they own the space and that space is not for the community. But we thought that that space was supposed to be for the community and it was supposed to give capacity building to the community."

As in India, organizations that took a more activist approach drew on networks that preceded government efforts to collaborate with them. For example, the Bar Hostesses' Empowerment and Support Project (BHESP) was an organization of sex workers that had been in existence since 1998. It had conducted HIV prevention with government funding but had also worked with feminist and human rights groups. It was part of a coalition of sex-worker–led organizations across Africa, the African Sex Workers' Alliance.[46] The coalition was run by an elected board, focused on legal aid and knowing your rights in the event of an arrest, and organized a yearly march and rally for the December 17 International Day to End Violence against Sex Workers. Its leaders were actively engaged in international networks of sex worker organizing, like the Network of Sex Work Projects, and traveled often to India and elsewhere in Asia as well as to other African countries for training and conferences. The coalition advocated for the rights of sex workers, including the decriminalization of sex work.

Sex workers, sexual minorities, and transgender groups with an activist bent approached South-South partnership in a distinct way from more biomedically focused organizations. Rather than drawing on Indian models of data management, they drew inspiration for activism. One activist, for example, said she learned to make demands on the state from activists in India. "We couldn't have sex workers volunteering for public clinics, and we saw that in India so we came and demanded it from NASCOP. Like, sex workers being directors and running their own things. We felt like the Indians do not even know how to speak English. Kenyan sex workers can speak English. That means we have a lot. We can run our own things. We have learned a lot, and they keep on empowering us all the time." Here, South-South partnership was less about adapting a technical model from a more advanced country: it was about mutual exchange across distinct contexts. Indeed, this interviewee challenged the hierarchy of Indian and Kenyan sex workers. Another activist had formed an organization of male sex workers after years of being an HIV peer educator. "You see the level of education of the sex workers in India is very different from Kenya, and you wonder why Kenya is not moving forward. . . . I formed [my organization] on what I saw from India," he told me. He had been to India several times to visit Indian sex worker organizations, and he was part of global networks of sex worker activism. "We also learnt from India that it is true that community intervention is very important to fight against HIV," he said.

Compared to Indian activism by sex workers, sexual minorities, and transgender people, these activist efforts unfolded at a smaller scale, without the framework of a national HIV prevention plan as a common target, platform, or anchor. But as changes in Kenyan AIDS policy shifted the balance in their favor—"all the money now is for key populations," one interviewee noted—these activists worked to influence its direction. For example, when NASCOP had become interested in working with sex workers, one activist said she had approached them and tried to explain that they were "not starting from zero." But there was no formal writing about existing efforts. With funding and support from the Gates Foundation, the Center for Global Public Health, NASCOP, and BHESP, they collaborated with Meena Seshu, a sex worker activist from India, to conduct a study on existing sex worker activism in Kenya.[47]

These moments—whether activists drawing inspiration from Indian collaborations as they advocated for their communities in Kenya or the documentation of existing sex worker activism by an Indian ally—marked openings in the travel of HIV prevention models across the global AIDS field. AIDS experts could use their funding and documentation skills to further the cause of sex worker activists who had long felt sidelined from the national AIDS response in Kenya. Within the global AIDS field, experts positioned Africa below India in a hierarchy of advancement and epidemic management. But the travel of the Indian model to Kenya simultaneously created spaces for connection, curiosity, mutual support and inspiration among activists across geographic lines.

CONTINENTAL SHIFTS

When I asked how effective efforts to replicate India's HIV prevention programs in Kenya had been, I mostly heard mixed reviews. "It has not peaked. It is not a friendly environment for sex workers," one staff member said about a drop-in center that had been set up that was, whenever I visited it, empty.

But another drop-in center I observed had taken root, with a warm, bois-terous environment and a regular community of visitors. This unevenness confirmed what many of my interviewees suggested: the circulation of best practices was never as simple as it looked on paper.[48]

Nevertheless, this chapter has uncovered how transnational exchanges unfolded in the context of a more fraught territory of hierarchy and solidarity. Within the global AIDS field, AIDS experts positioned India as an effective model that could be circulated, evoking a colonial and postcolonial legacy of adapting "advanced" Indian models to African contexts. These hierarchies were anchored by ideas of technical and political progress and sexual culture that evoked deep-seated racialized hierarchies. But these hierarchies were taken up in different ways. For some, they reinforced the need for Indian HIV prevention strategies in Kenya. For others, they demonstrated the irrelevance of Indian approaches to the Kenyan epidemic. They also yielded a variety of programmatic directions. Some organizations took from the Indian model a new individualized approach to planning and monitoring. Others took an approach to activism that demanded inclusion in state programs and prioritized grassroots leadership.

The variety of discourses on Africa in the Indian (and African) imagi-nation within AIDS programs suggests that the response to the AIDS crisis could not be separated from the political and symbolic relationships be-tween the two countries that anchored their positions in the global AIDS field. Feminist historian Isabel Hofmeyer[49] highlights two Indian nationalist discourses about Africa—one in which Africa stood in solidarity with India against British colonization and an older one in which India found its limits in its African "others." Thus, "Africa functions as a shorthand for all that is backward. Africa becomes one of India's nightmare pasts that it is trying to escape. As the colony was to the metropolis, so Africa is to India: belated, backward, haunting."[50] Traces of both of these discourses surface within AIDS programs across India and Kenya. Visions of collaboration, the sharing of best practices, and uniting against a devastating crisis operated alongside discourses on hierarchical difference, competition, and solidarity, with which Indian and Kenyan experts had to contend.

8 | AFTER AIDS

EXPERTS INCREASINGLY DISCUSS the end of AIDS.[1] But UNAIDS officials insist that AIDS is not over.[2] In 2016, the UN resolved to end the AIDS epidemic by 2030, but by 2018 Michel Sidibé, director of UNAIDS, warned that the world was falling off track to meet this goal.[3] Funds and energy seemed to be drying up for the AIDS response. AIDS no longer holds the claim on the global attention it once did. This shift is built into the logic and definition of crisis. As the editors of a recent volume note, "By definition, crisis is exception. . . . a crisis is not meant to last."[4] Yet, they point out, the crisis has not ended; it has only been redistributed.[5] Even as everyday crises of life with HIV unfold every day all over the world, even as AIDS-related illnesses are the leading cause of death for women between the ages of fifteen and forty-nine globally,[6] even as 1.7 million people newly seroconverted in 2018,[7] amid the shifting tides of public discourse, the global AIDS crisis is over.

When I arrived in India in 2012, AIDS experts tended to talk about the height of the crisis in the past tense. Some even sounded nostalgic. The Gates Foundation was just beginning to hand over its programs to state agencies.[8] In 2014, the Department of AIDS Control, which since 2009 had bureaucratically separated AIDS from other diseases, merged with the Ministry of Health and Family Welfare.[9] AIDS was no longer an exceptional crisis that required exceptional administrative means to control. In Kenya, the atmosphere was strikingly different. Interviewees spoke of sustained effort but frustratingly uneven progress. Even government documents spoke of HIV prevalence rates that were "stabilizing," but with "significant challenges ahead."[10]

There was no particular reason to believe India would avert its looming AIDS epidemic. In 1986, when physicians documented India's first known case of HIV,[11] Indian life expectancy was fifty-six years,[12] and, except for in a few states,[13] the majority of deaths in the country resulted from communicable diseases.[14] India's health infrastructure has always grappled with the general conditions of poverty and inequality, alongside its overstretched bureaucracy. India was one of the last countries in the world to eradicate polio.[15] Even when there is progress on health indicators, absolute impact remains high. The WHO estimates, for example, that India accounts for 15% of all maternal deaths in the world.[16] On top of these limitations to the public health system was the fact that AIDS is largely a sexually transmitted disease. The criminalization of sex workers, sexual minorities, and transgender people made even basic conversations about HIV prevention difficult to imagine.

Given this context, at least according to the numbers, India's AIDS response was an unlikely success. With an estimated 2.1 million people living with HIV in 2017,[17] India still has one of the world's largest AIDS epidemics, but since a peak in 1995, the number of new HIV cases every year declined by 85% by 2017, to around 88,000.[18] A relatively low 0.22% of Indians are estimated to be HIV positive.[19] In 2015, halting and reversing the AIDS epidemic was one of the few Millennium Development Goals India was considered to have met.[20] India is "the pharmacy of the world," producing nearly 85% of the generic AIDS drugs used globally.[21] One World Bank report presents the Indian sex worker community response to HIV as "one of the most impressive in the world."[22] NACO's website claims that "India's AIDS Control Programme is globally acclaimed as a success story."[23] "India is the biggest success story in the world when it comes to AIDS control," said Sujata Rao, the former director of NACO, in a news interview on World AIDS Day 2015. "Just humane interventions and home-grown strategies did it for us in a society that is so closed that we were asked to air condom ads after 11pm when children were asleep."[24]

These accounts of success and failure, of risk and disaster, suggest that

> CHANGES HOW THE
STATE RELATES TO
THEIR CITIZENS

the management of national crisis never occurs in a vacuum. Rather, states define and respond to crisis within a global field. The AIDS crisis pushed the Indian state to navigate a global order. Risk and success were defined in relation to Africa and the West. A 2015 news article notes that "India, with its vast swathes of densely populated, unhygienic living quarters, crippling poverty and malnutrition was widely believed then [in the 1990s] to be the next sub-Saharan Africa in terms of the sheer numbers and spread of AIDS. As yet another World AIDS Day is observed, India can afford to look back with some satisfaction at its AIDS control programme."[25]

These navigations of the global AIDS field intersected with the state's relationship to a shifting and uneven political terrain within India. Under pressure to handle globally circulating warnings of India's unique risk, Indian state officials brutally targeted women in sex work in particular as the source of risk. But as India's AIDS crisis increasingly became a global problem and attracted global donor funding, crisis management created a terrain on which sex workers, sexual minorities, and transgender people could articulate new political claims and new ways of embodying and practicing sexuality. India's AIDS response—and its circulation to Kenya and elsewhere—took shape within hybrid, relatively autonomous pockets within the state,[26] within which national state agencies, transnational donors, and local sex worker, sexual minority, and transgender groups were uniquely interdependent. Ultimately, this book shows how global crisis generates an uneven terrain that can yield sometimes unexpected political openings and even transnational connections, openings within which political claims around gender and sexuality can be redefined.[27]

In making this argument, I do not intend to suggest that AIDS programs in India were perfectly successful. Activists continue to challenge the logic of the crisis's end and puncture the story of AIDS as an unequivocal success. Rather than assessing the success of AIDS interventions, the goal of this book has been to understand the political implications of the AIDS crisis for the relationships between state and society within a shifting global context, in particular for the sex workers, sexual minorities, and transgender people HIV prevention programs target. Narratives of decline, co-optation, and absorption are common in many of my interviewees' accounts of AIDS activism. Yet while studies have rightly pointed to the shortsightedness of donor-funded state AIDS programs in India and argued that they depoliticize sexuality,[28] this book finds that AIDS interventions also unexpectedly became sites for experimentation, solidarity, care, the formation of citizenship, and even new transnational connections. In doing so, I hope to recover the complexities of sexual and political life, and even moments of transformation and joy, in contexts of criminalization, disease, and biomedical surveillance.[29]

What happens to those who outlive a crisis? For millions of people living with HIV, and for the sex workers, sexual minorities, and transgender people who were swept into a massive global crisis response, the end of AIDS is a complicated prospect. For many, it means their concerns have been forgotten, funding for the programs they depend on slashed. For some of those I came to know over the course of my research, however, the slowing of the AIDS response was a relief. "We have *survived* HIV funding," one activist corrected me, when I asked how they had used HIV funds. The end of HIV meant less medical surveillance and more holistic and democratic possibilities for articulating sexual identity.[30] This was especially true for middle-class, dominant-caste sexual minorities and transgender people, who had seen dramatic legal and social shifts in the two decades since the beginning of the AIDS response. For others, it meant the return of a status quo of exploitation, marginalization, and state violence. Without the crisis to lend national urgency to their claims, and without the logistical resources HIV prevention NGOs provided, they would join the chorus of those struggling for basic survival and recognition in contemporary India.

Crises are, by definition, temporary. The more mundane circumstances of poverty or dispossession often do not attain the same urgency as a crisis response.[31] Craig Calhoun notes that the idea of the *emergency* serves to "represent as sudden, unpredictable, and short-term what are usually gradually developing, predictable, and enduring clusters of events and interactions."[32] Seen in this light, AIDS becomes a temporary emergency rather than a long-term symptom of social transformations. This transience was not necessarily a surprise to those at the heart of the AIDS response in India. When I interviewed him in 2013, one NGO manager noted,

> [It] is only a matter of time; you'll be a victim of your own success. The minute you bring [HIV] down to zero, which we want to, you'll not be funded, no one will care about you, you'll be back to being the pariah of society which we'll find new ways to target. That's how women have

always been used. . . . If a situation comes, if they have to save their skin, they drop these women like hot potatoes. That's the reality. Nobody will care for you; there will be no KHPT, no Avahan, BMGF [Bill and Melinda Gates Foundation], or government willing to look at you. You have to stand on your own feet.

The interview captured the contradictions of the AIDS crisis. It created a temporary moment of recognition, a brief opening, but once the risk had passed, the moment would too. When I returned to Bangalore in 2015, two years after my fieldwork, this prediction had largely come true. KHPT, which had been set up to help manage the AIDS response in Karnataka, was engaged in projects on new topics, such as orphans and vulnerable children and maternal and child health. The state agency for AIDS prevention was continuing to fund programs, but on a much smaller budget. Sex workers, sexual minorities, and transgender people who had come to rely on HIV prevention work for part of their income had not been paid in almost a year because of funding delays. Some drop-in centers I had once visited to find full of people dancing to movie songs, watching TV, and taking naps were empty, and people spoke with wistful nostalgia about the days when there was tea and biscuits, or even biryani. Many had gone back to their old lives and workplaces. Meanwhile, a new right-wing government seemed uninterested in HIV prevention and was repressing NGOs that were critical of the state, especially if they received international funding.[33]

These changes suggested the conditionality of the forms of citizenship the AIDS crisis offered to its at-risk citizens. Sex workers, sexual minorities, and transgender people were incorporated partially into state programs, so long as they posed a risk to the nation, but other aspects of sexual regulation remained untouched. A legal activist I interviewed in Delhi pointed out:

Internationally HIV has fallen off the map, and you see the effects of it domestically. And the fact that all NACO reports are saying there's been a dramatic decline, and the latest figures say that HIV national prevalence among sex workers is about 2.7%, so it's less than 5%, which means that it's no longer even a concentrated epidemic. So you can say look, sex workers have obviously contributed the most to HIV control, but then what? . . . that's the other problem with what's happened in India. . . . it's not discussed very often, but it is something we are trying to deal with. The whole discourse [that] you will be able to control HIV, protect rights, have policy reforms, protect the rights of sex workers. India's managed to contain HIV without reforming sex work law.

The end of the global AIDS crisis thus had mixed effects for the social movements that had formed around it. It had transformed the possibilities, but only temporarily. At first, without the urgency of HIV prevention on their side, activists had fewer tools in their arsenal to reform laws regulating sexuality. When the Ministry of Women and Child Development proposed amendments to the ITPA in 2013 that sought to criminalize sex work, an interviewee noted, "There is no mobilization now." In 2013, in *Suresh Kumar Koushal and Another v. Naz Foundation and Others*,[34] the Supreme Court overturned the Delhi High Court's 2009 judgment overturning Section 377's application to homosexuality, effectively recriminalizing gay sex. This time, arguments about HIV prevention played a much less prominent role than they had in the 2009 deliberations.[35] As AIDS programs were merged with other Ministry of Health departments, one activist in Delhi described it as "going back a hundred steps." With AIDS no longer a focus of government and public attention, sex worker, sexual minority, and transgender citizenship again seemed to be in question. The hybrid spaces of the AIDS response were slowly being dismantled, and the political assertions built on the AIDS response no longer carried the same force.

To some extent, forms of citizenship articulated in the time of the AIDS crisis could not be undone. Over the course of three decades, the relationships between sex worker groups and the state had undergone significant shifts. In 2012, in the aftermath of the notorious Delhi gang rape, as Parliament deliberated a Criminal Law Amendment Bill that would define prostitution as a form of sexual exploitation, the reaction from sex worker networks was almost immediate. Protests took shape within a day all over the country, and the Verma Commission, on whose report the bill was based, issued a clarification noting that the definition did not apply to those who engaged in prostitution "of their own free will."[36] In 2013, Parliament passed the act with the word *prostitution* omitted altogether. The Verma Commission had consulted sex worker groups in the preparation of the report, and sex workers were accommodated after they protested the outcome. In 2018, the

Lok Sabha, the Indian Parliament's lower house, passed an Anti-Trafficking Bill that, in furthering opportunities for state violence against sex workers without addressing the roots of sex trafficking, drew critique from sex worker activists. Though the bill's passage presented a significant setback, the way the debate unfolded over the bill suggested that sex workers were no longer relegated to the margins of public discourse. Representatives from the National Network of Sex Workers opposed the bill, with the support of the well-known Congress politician Shashi Tharoor, and were quoted in the media with their critiques.[37] Nevertheless, the circularity of the debate, Prabha Kotiswaran points out, underscored that "the dial on sex work has barely moved."[38]

In the years after the height of the global AIDS crisis, sexual minority and transgender politics made major legal gains, far beyond the early steps that AIDS organizations had initiated. After five years of persistent legal activism and public pressure, in the 2018 *Navtej Singh Johar and Others v. Union of India* judgment,[39] the Supreme Court ruled that Section 377 of the Indian Penal Code was unconstitutional in criminalizing consensual same-sex relationships. The judgment was celebrated all over the world and solidified a palpable shift in the visibility of queer politics in India. The judgment relied much less on AIDS-related arguments than the 2009 ruling, instead focusing on individual self-determination, antidiscrimination, and universal citizenship. The 2014 *National Legal Services Authority v. Union of India and Others* Supreme Court judgment declared transgender people a "third gender" with fundamental constitutional rights, including the right to reservations as a "backward" class.[40] The 2019 Transgender Persons (Protection of Rights) Bill, which passed in the Lok Sabha in July, attempted to put the ruling into practice. But it faced bitter opposition from transgender rights groups, who argued that the bill had not been adequately debated or discussed by transgender groups, that it failed to address the complexity of discrimination and exclusion transgender people face, and that it placed new medical and juridical restrictions on the identification of transgender people that would inadvertently increase the policing and regulation of transgender people's lives.

In 2020, when a new crisis rendered those who rely on public spaces for livelihood and intimacy particularly vulnerable—including sex workers, sexual minorities, and transgender people—the organizational structure and activist networks this book has traced mobilized around a new cause.

Activists worked to deliver emergency food rations and mental health counseling. When a group of medical researchers at Harvard and Yale published a study recommending that Indian red-light districts be closed to stop COVID-19, the National Network of Sex Workers published a scathing and witty critique, while a letter signed by prominent activists, lawyers, and health officials received a response from both medical schools the same day.[41] That the researchers were subject to not only immediate protest but also ridicule suggests that sex workers could not be detained or threatened because of sexual panic in the face of a deadly virus, as they had been in 1986.

Ultimately, the relationship between sexual minority, sex worker, and transgender groups and the state remains an inconclusive and fraught terrain. The global AIDS crisis lent temporary urgency to activists' efforts; their demands were heard, if only in the name of managing risk, and supported by public health agencies within the state. "After" the crisis, sex worker, sexual minority, and transgender groups engaged the state on a different footing. They were less insulated from the shifting terrain of democratic politics; they were more reliant on the diverse coalitions they had been able to build outside of state institutions and donor funding. Sexual minority and transgender groups, with their growing global support, fared better in this new landscape than sex worker groups, especially when faced with opposition from globally funded anti-prostitution advocates.[42]

In Kenya, the struggle also played out unevenly. Kenya has seen growing activism from sex workers, sexual minorities, and transgender people,[43] including the continued work of the Kenya Sex Workers' Alliance and its participation in regional and transnational sex worker networks. In 2016, John Mathenge, the founder of Health Options for Young Men on HIV/AIDS/STI (HOYMAS), an HIV prevention NGO for male sex workers, along with several other activists from LGBTQ organizations, filed two petitions in the High Court challenging the criminalization of homosexuality on the grounds of the rights to dignity, nondiscrimination, and health. In 2019, the petitions were rejected.[44] I remembered what an interviewee told me in 2013, "We use the HIV platform to advocate for other rights. That is the platform in Kenya that people use, everyone . . . everyone, [they] are all being protected by HIV/AIDS. . . . There's a lot more than HIV . . . [but] NASCOP is the only platform that we as key populations can hide in."

THE POLITICS OF CRISIS

AIDS has been defined as a crisis. Many other issues are not. There is no cross-cutting UN agency dedicated specifically to addressing the relationships between land grabs that dispossess peasants, droughts that increase the numbers of poor migrants seeking precarious employment in Indian cities, patriarchal systems that render sexual minorities and transgender people socially and economically exploitable, and gentrification of public spaces that lead to new waves of police violence against those who earn their livelihood through sex. There is not even a UN agency to address LGBTQ rights.[45] But once sex workers and men who have sex with men were designated at risk of HIV, they had a new point of access to the state. They were now a significant force in fighting a global crisis. The progress of nations in fighting AIDS is assessed and compared. Billions of dollars have been spent on the cause.

The response to the AIDS crisis has brought issues that were once marginal onto the global agenda. Risk management made invisible struggles, the everyday crises of being criminalized on the basis of sexuality, significant within a global field. Before AIDS, the fact that landlords would not agree to rent rooms to sex workers and their children, or that transgender women were beaten and harassed by police officers, did not receive urgent attention. It took activism to bring these everyday crises within the purview of what the state, donors, and public health researchers understood to be an appropriate AIDS response. Activists drew on their existing political alliances and forged new ones, leveraging the resources devoted to the crisis to redefine the crisis response in ways that would address its structural roots. Ultimately, they altered the definition of crisis, refocusing it on long-term social and economic exclusions.

By focusing on how crisis was defined and contested in India and then repurposed in Kenya, this book offers insights on the paradoxes of contemporary humanitarianism. "In contemporary societies," the anthropologist Didier Fassin writes, "where inequalities have reached an unprecedented level, humanitarianism elicits the fantasy of a global moral community that may still be viable and the expectation that solidarity may have redeeming powers."[46] Nicola Mai and Elizabeth Bernstein show how sexual humanitarianism tethers these fantasies of rescue to sexual politics.[47] Crisis gives the impression of suffering as a temporary aberration and, as such, as something that can be rectified. Patriarchy, capitalism, and transphobia feel overwhelm-ing; AIDS programs with sex workers feel more manageable. They can be planned and assessed; concrete results can be measured and compared. Crisis response, in this way, is a template for various forms of global intervention. In a contradictory way, being affected by a crisis can be a ticket to resources otherwise unavailable to the majority of people exploited or excluded by capitalist processes. If this book suggests that crises can create unexpected gains, it is only because life outside crisis is often already unlivable.

By centering the political implications of crisis, and the relationships be-tween global crises and the everyday crises that underpin them, this book has suggested a multiscalar approach to studying global fields. Sociologists who study global fields often focus on global institutions, or on nation-states in the global field; they turn less often to the relationships between national states and local social movements. This book has worked to connect scholarship on the state and society with scholarship on global fields. It has also worked to position India, as a postcolonial nation-state, within a more multidimensional field of struggle—not just engaged in a North-South binary of top-down global institutions and local resistance but also involved in repositioning itself in the world order as an emerging power. In tracing the circulation of AIDS expertise from India to Kenya, this book has shown how South-South relationships can both reproduce hierarchies among nations and provide opportunities for reworking them.

By analyzing the production of and contestation over crisis, this book has offered ways of thinking about when and why certain issues reach crisis proportions and how existing social movements shape the response. The Indian crisis did not emerge solely from state agencies' response to the needs of its citizens. It was produced and debated within a global AIDS field. What counts as a crisis, who is affected by it, and what needs to be done to stop it can occasion intense political struggle. The uncertainty of crisis also may entail a bitter set of trade-offs for social movements. They must engage the state and transnational donors to survive, even if it means surveillance, co-optation, and political concessions. These spaces of concrete messiness in engaging the state have long been a topic of feminist inquiry,[48] but crisis raises the stakes.

The global AIDS response is one example of how global crises are man-aged by a complex of actors that includes states, global governance institu-tions, and powerful private donors. In the context of widespread state failure, the Gates Foundation has already pledged US$1.75 billion to the COVID-19 response. Despite Bill Gates's insistence that the Foundation can only serve as a "stopgap" or "catalyst,"[49] the Gates Foundation wields tremendous influence over global health. Though increasingly prioritizing agriculture, the Gates Foundation spent US$1.5 billion on global health programs in 2019 alone,[50] and it is second only to the US government in its contributions to the WHO, accounting for up 12% of the WHO's budget.[51] Scholars and activists have challenged the Gates Foundation's brand of philanthro-capitalism, including its emphasis on technological fixes and quick innovations, its insistence on corporate involvement in public health, and its unaccountable role in setting priorities for the global health agenda.[52] All these tendencies were in evidence in the Gates Foundation's Avahan program in India, and many of my interviewees, including state officials, NGOs, and activists, were critical of its role. At the same time, they knew there was no avoiding the Gates Foundation. This book suggests that those most successful in sustaining their autonomy operated on the terrain of the global AIDS field in nimble and creative ways, building both global and local alliances to serve as a counterweight to the Foundation's imperatives.

The politics of crisis this book has traced extend beyond public health. After the notorious Delhi gang rape in 2012, for example, sexual violence in India newly emerged as a crisis. Once a persistent, quietly tolerated feature of everyday life, sexual violence became an epidemic of urgent concern.[53] As protests erupted all over the country and India's levels of sexual violence attracted global attention, a well-established feminist movement with long experience working to end sexual violence shaped the state's response. The involvement of these feminist groups counteracted, at least partly, the tendency for a more nativist and morally conservative reaction to the rape. Global crisis intersected with local political articulations to create an opening for legal change.[54] Crises both further conditions of exclusion and create possibilities for renegotiating them.

LIFE AFTER RISK

This book is concerned with how the global AIDS crisis reshaped the lives of sex workers, sexual minorities, and transgender people in everyday ways. In 2015, when I visited Preethi, a transgender woman I had gotten to know well during fieldwork, she was no longer working in HIV prevention. The NGO office was much less active than it had been before. "It's not like before—only staff come, no one from the community. It's really sad to see now. I wanted to go to the office the other day when I heard it was open, but I didn't have time. . . . They have no funds. They're saying it will close soon. They don't call us for events anymore. They did a protest, and I would have gone, but they didn't come to tell me."

In 2017, when I visited Preethi again, she proudly showed me a letter of employment for a local charity. An NGO she knew through her old connections when she had worked as an HIV peer educator had provided her with job training. On a day-to-day basis, her main sources of support were her closest friends, her neighbors, and the relatives who occasionally came to visit. Preethi largely felt left behind by HIV prevention spaces that had once played a role in her life. But the connections and friendships she had formed during the AIDS crisis had become one more resource she could leverage in seeking employment.

When I called Sita, a cisgender woman sex worker, in 2015 to ask how she was doing, she said she now earned her income from a combination of agricultural day labor and sex work. A few days later I met her at the bus stop in her town. She arrived walking briskly. She told me she had some work to do at the courthouse. She had been involved in a property dispute for two years now, and she was waiting for the police case to come through against an abusive relative. Sita held a brown paper envelope full of documents related to the property dispute. We walked in, and she sat across from a lawyer with a distant manner. Sita smiled, said hello, and asked when the court date would be. The lawyer said someone else had to set it, so we should wait. In the meantime, Sita sat patiently, chatting with everyone who came in and out. Then Sita turned back to the task. "You said to bring these documents," she said, pulling them out. The lawyer looked through them slowly and distractedly, before nodding and turning back to another pile of documents. We went upstairs, and Sita nearly accosted the wiry man responsible. Against his languid protests, she asked him over and over until he scribbled a date down on her envelope. Later that afternoon, I asked Sita if she thought working in a sex worker organization had made any difference in her life. "One thing is that before, I didn't used to be able to talk like this," she said. "Like how I was going around in the courthouse, talking to everyone." In 2017, when I visited Sita, she had opened a vegetable stall in her town market.

Sita had spent her life working—as a child in a factory, as a young adult in sex work, then as an HIV prevention peer educator, then as an activist, then as an agricultural laborer, then as a street vendor. Many aspects of her life had not changed. But at thirty-two, she already had a son who was entering engineering college, a partner she was happy with, and a number of friends in her neighborhood. The AIDS crisis had not given Sita these openings to material security and social solidarity. She was involved in Dalit activism and in a women's self-help group in her community, and these spaces had shaped her in fundamental ways. She had taught herself to read and write using her son's school texts and practiced every day in a small cardboard-bound note-book. But her involvement in HIV prevention had offered Sita new avenues to navigating the state. She had learned, as she put it, to talk, "Wherever I went, I didn't used to talk bravely. That's the first point. I wasn't able to talk bravely. I hadn't learned how to talk properly. Now I always talk boldly, whether it's to the police, or thugs, it could be anyone, no problem. I have the strength now to ask what's going on. Once you have courage, then no matter where you are, you can live." This learning to talk was an unexpected side effect of the massive HIV prevention effort in India. A global crisis had opened up a new way of articulating solidarity with other sex workers and navigating the everyday hassles of accessing welfare as a marginalized woman.

As a woman and a sex worker, poor and Dalit, Sita faced brutal circum-stances in her everyday life. The AIDS crisis had not particularly changed these conditions. It had treated them as exceptional, as factors to be dealt with so long as Sita posed a risk to the general population. Yet there were some lasting changes in the aftermath of crisis. AIDS forced the state and donors to provide some small openings for staking collective claims. Some of these solidarities, formal or informal, lasted beyond the crisis. And they occasioned some individual transformations that prepared Sita, in her everyday life, to navigate the state. This book has marked the contradictions of a state that needed the risk of catastrophic crisis to consider the claims of criminalized citizens and to confront its own fraught legacies of regulating sexuality.

Acknowledgments

This project has benefited from extraordinary mentorship and intellectual generosity. Raka Ray combines a path-breaking commitment to fostering transnational feminist scholarship in sociology with theoretical rigor and ethnographic savvy. She was there through every twist and turn of this project, from initial inchoate proposal drafts to frantic Skype calls in the midst of fieldwork, and throughout my long, slow process of finding my voice as an academic. Peter Evans supported my scholarly formation from the very beginning, and pushed me to find room for intellectual optimism and to think comparatively and globally about the dynamics of neoliberal globalization. Gillian Hart not only helped me work through the complexities of fieldwork but also played a key role in shaping my understanding of political struggle and transnational method. Lawrence Cohen's enthusiasm and intellectual expansiveness made for wonderful conversations and inspired me to think more creatively about my material. I was lucky to learn from Michael Burawoy about the craft of teaching. His faith in me made me feel I belong in sociology when, many times, I myself did not believe it, and his commitment to social theory is a constant reminder of the gifts of a thinking life. I am also grateful to Ann Swidler, who, through many generous conversations, helped me get to the heart of what mattered about my project, and Marion Fourcade, whose intellectual rigor and clarity has often pushed me to sharpen my ideas. Several other Berkeley faculty members have played crucial roles in the intellectual journey that led to this book, among them Paola Bacchetta, Aihwa Ong, Cihan Tugal, and Laura Enriquez, and I am deeply grateful to them all.

At Berkeley, I benefited from the presence of a transformative community of gender scholars who continue to be a source of inspiration. Raka Ray's dissertation group and the Gender and Sexuality Workshop—among them Katherine Maich, Carter Koppelman, Louise Ly, Joy Hightower, Gillian Gualtieri, Tara Gonsalves, Jason Ferguson, Kate Mason, Abigail Andrews, and Jennifer Carlson—suffered through early iterations of key chapters at various points, and Kimberly Kay Hoang's support helped move this project from dissertation to book.

My early exposure to the politics of AIDS would not have been possible without my mentors at Brown University and in Durban, South Africa—in particular, Mark Lurie, Jenni Smit, Zonke Mabude, and Letitia Rambally. Catherine Burns has warmly and generously supported my work. I also thank Mark Hunter for an illuminating early conversation.

For their generous support of me and my work and willingness to help me make connections, I would like to thank Shubha Chacko, Akkai Padmashali, Sundar Sundararaman, Parinita Bhattacharjee, Meena Seshu, Smarajit Jana, Benoy Peter, and Shakun Doundiyakhed. Meeting Shubha Chacko and Subadra Panchanadeswaran has been one of the greatest gifts of doing this project, and my collaboration and friendship with them continues to sustain me. In particular, I thank Shubha for hosting and feeding me for weeks on end, for being the best of travel companions, and for advice and solidarity throughout my project. I would also like to thank Priya Prabhu, Sravanthi Dasari, Kannan, and Shyam for their support, and in particular Priya, Kannan, and Jayashree for their meticulous transcription work and Sakshi for thoughtful research assistance. In Bangalore, I benefited from conversations with a vibrant community of scholars, including Hemangini Gupta, Carol Upadhya, Supriya Roychowdhury, Smriti Srinivas, Kanthi Krishnamurthy, and Manisha Anantharaman. Kiran Keshavamurthy has not only been a wonderful friend but also hosted me in Kolkata during my fieldwork, and Joyojeet Pal has made me laugh and helped me figure things out. I would like to thank Amita Baviskar for insightful conversations at key points. I draw inspiration from brilliant scholars of sex work and sexuality in India who have engaged with my work, including Prabha

Kotiswaran, Svati Shah, Kimberly Walters, Vibhuti Ramachandran, Chaitanya Lakkimsetti, Simanti Dasgupta, Mirna Guha, Pankhuri Agarwal, and Shakthi Nataraj.

Jocelyn Viterna, Jyoti Puri, and Ulka Anjaria read the entire manuscript and gave me the kind of brilliant, sharp, and transformative feedback I could not have imagined possible. My thanks to Carina Ray, Elizabeth Ferry, and Cheryl Hansen for their support in organizing my book manuscript workshop, and to Ann Ward and Sanchita Dasgupta for their meticulous notetaking. I am grateful to the brilliant sociologists of South Asia who have read and debated parts of my work with me—Smitha Radhakrishnan, Poulami Roychowdhury, Rina Agarwala, Paromita Sanyal, Fareen Parvez, Michael Levien, Patrick Heller, and Rajesh Veeraraghavan. Presentations at the Center for the Study of Culture and Society, the Bangalore Research Network, the South Asia by the Bay conference, Bowdoin College, Wheaton College, Boston University, the Harvard University Transnational Studies Initiative, the Watson Institute at Brown University, and the wonderful workshop on Interdisciplinary Conversations on Sex Work in India have helped me to sharpen the ideas in this book at various points. My thanks to Tejaswini Niranjana, Nitya Vasudevan, Hemangini Gupta, Anjali Arondekar, Puneeta Kala, Sanchita Saxena, Sridevi Prasad, Jay Sosa, Katherine Mason, Joseph Harris, Jocelyn Viterna, Peggy Levitt, Patrick Heller, Prabha Kotiswaran, and Shakthi Nataraj for making these conversations possible. Funding from the Social Science Research Council and a workshop facilitated by Ruth Toulson and Julia Phillips Cohen supported the fieldwork for this project, along with funding from the National Science Foundation and the Tomberg Research Funds and Norman Grant at Brandeis University. I also benefited from the American Institute of Indian Studies Dissertation into Book Workshop, facilitated by Geraldine Forbes and Ron Herring, and in particular from brilliant comments on my proposal from Venera Khalikova, and insightful feedback and encouragement from Navyug Gill and Lipika Kamra.

At Brandeis, my colleagues Siri Suh, Patricia Alvarez Astacio, Derron Wallace, Mike Strand, Sara Shostak, Karen Hansen, Wendy Cadge, Carmen Sirianni, Laura Miller, Peter Conrad, Cheryl Hansen, Lauren Jordahl, Sarah Mayorga, Brian Horton, Shoniqua Roach, V Varun Chaudhury, Yuri Doolan, Jon Anjaria, Ulka Anjaria, Carina Ray, Elizabeth Ferry, Hannah Muller, Jeffrey Lenowitz, Sarah Lamb, Harleen Singh, Sue Lanser, and Faith Smith, among many others, have brought me intellectual and personal sustenance. I am grateful to Marcela Maxfield at Stanford University Press for her faith in my work from the very beginning and her efficient and thoughtful engagement in my project, and to Sunna Juhn, Jessica Ling, Stephanie Adams, Athena Lakri, and the rest of the team for making the process seamless.

When I was a graduate student, I often read the acknowledgments in books, looking for traces of the long path to writing them. My journey through writing has posed its share of small disasters. A luminous community of friends and family has sustained me with dinners and late-into-the-night conversations, visited me and traveled with me during fieldwork, celebrated milestones, took me shopping when I lost all my belongings in a house fire, brought dinner when I was solo parenting and teaching at the same time, checked in on me from afar, and sent groceries and cheered me up with Zoom calls when I was diagnosed with COVID-19 a few weeks before I was due to submit my manuscript (and again a second time six months later!). I would not have survived my PhD, or life after it, without the support and love of Louise Ly, Katy Fox-Hodess, and Zachary Levenson, who have talked me through both the ideas in this book and the angst of writing it. Berkeley friends Elizabeth Pearson, Carter Koppelman, Carlos Bustamante, Sunmin Kim, Sujin Eom, Herbert Docena, Rebecca Elliott, Margaret Frye, Pablo Gaston, Katherine Maich, Tara Gonsalves, Jason Ferguson, Preeti Shekar, and Harsha Mallajosyula have helped me find my way as an academic. Kareem Khubchandani has read parts of this book more carefully than I have and is the auntie and sister I never knew I needed, and Dwai Banerjee has failed to distract me several times during writing sessions at coffee shops; thank you for being my Boston auntie family. I thank Ana Villareal, Patricia Alvarez Astacio, Siri Suh, Saida Grundy, Laura Nelson, Elena Shih, Jeffrey Lenowitz, Hande Inanc, Jon Anjaria, Ulka Anjaria, Emmerich Davies, Joseph Harris, Poulami Roychowdhury, and Ghassan Moussawi for making the task of being a junior scholar much less daunting. For years, Julia Chuang has been an off-duty therapist and intellectual inspiration rolled into one. Without Smitha Radhakrishnan's friendship and the brilliant example of creativity and scholarship she sets, I would probably not be a (dancing) sociologist. The members of the Massachusetts Sex Worker Ally Network have helped me find political meaning and direction in Boston.

My oldest friends, Kristen Chin, Nadia Lambek, Ceara O'Leary, Nayla Khoury, Smitha Khorana, Alexis Walker, Mary Greene, Sophia Warshall, Si-yuan Xie, Daphne Schatzberg, Praveen Basaviah, Manu Lohiya, Layli Uddin, Bali Kumar, Mohini Venkatesh, Roopa Chari, Andrew DeBenedictis, Pooja Sripad, Abhishek Sripad, Vijay Umapathy, and Shalu Umapathy have been my anchors, among many others. This book would not have been written without the brilliant and loving people who have cared for my child—among them Thaty Oliveira, Bridget Dixon, Naseem Anjaria, Marin Sewell and Jillian McVey. My in-laws, Susan Montgomery, Michael Williams, Marj Montgomery, and Michael Shea, have stepped in at several moments with crucial support and endless thoughtfulness. My Harohalli, Kurpad, and Andover uncles, aunties, and cousins, biological and not, in the US and India, have sustained me and nourished me over these years. In particular, I am grateful to my Bangalore relatives who have cared for me during fieldwork, and to Srinivas Raju, who not only picked me up from the airport on every visit without fail but also talked with me about fieldwork and helped me find my way.

My parents, Jyothi and Harohalli Vijayakumar, are the ones who taught me what I needed to know to be a sociologist. Though unfamiliar with the world of academia, they set an example with their compassionate interest in others, their adventurousness, their passion for learning, their brilliant philosophical minds, and their intuitive sense of justice. Over the course of this project, they not only supported me unconditionally in too many ways to document but also traveled with me during parts of my fieldwork. Nandini Vijayakumar is my younger sister, but she has often been the one with the maturity, wisdom, faith, and goodness to guide me through rough waters. Joshua Williams has read every word of this manuscript and walked along-side me on every step of its making; he is my refuge, my source of strength and safety and laughter, my brilliant friend. Kavi has endured this book's writing with remarkable patience. He has transformed me, and brought me joy and purpose.

I cannot name several of the people who were most important to the development of this project to protect their anonymity. They might not read this book, or agree with what it says, but I hope I have been able to capture their courage, creativity, and generosity in some small way.

Appendixes

APPENDIX 1. Detailed are the duration, budget, and main components for four phases of Indian AIDS policy from 1992 to 2017.
SOURCE: National AIDS Control Organization (NACO) documents, compiled by author.

PHASE	DURATION	BUDGET[1]	MAIN PRIORITIES/STRATEGIES[2]
NACP I (National AIDS Control Programme I)	1992–1999	$113 million	• Strengthening management capacity for HIV/AIDS prevention and control through the formation and support of organizational structures at the national and state levels • Promoting public awareness and community support for AIDS prevention (through TV and radio, private advertising, NGOs, and the health system) • Improving blood safety • Building surveillance and clinical management capacity • Controlling sexually transmitted diseases
NACP II	1999–2006	$460 million	• Prevention of further spread of the disease (including awareness, condom promotion, STD control, blood safety, and reinforcing traditional Indian moral values) • Creating an enabling socioeconomic environment so that all sections of population can protect themselves from the infection and so families and communities can provide care and support to people living with HIV/AIDS • Improving services for the care of people living with AIDS

NACP III	2007–2012	$2.5 billion	• Preventing new infections in high-risk groups and general population (70% of the budget) • Providing greater care, support, and treatment to larger numbers of people living with HIV/AIDS • Strengthening the infrastructure, systems, and human resources for scaling up prevention, care, support, and treatment programs at the district, state, and national level • Strengthening the nationwide Strategic Information Management System
NACP IV	2012–2017	$2.1 billion	• Intensifying and consolidating prevention services, with a focus on high-risk groups and vulnerable populations • Increasing access and promoting comprehensive care, support, and treatment • Expanding IEC services for general population and high-risk groups with a focus on behavior change and demand generation • Building capacities at national, state, district, and facility levels • Strengthening Strategic Information Management Systems

1. These budget numbers for NACP I, II, and III come from a 2010 NACO summary report. Because of continual revisions of budget estimates, documents from various stages of the NACP report have different budget numbers; for example, the World Bank report on NACP II reports a budget of $433 million, not $460 million. There are also changes in reports of expenditure; for example, a 2003 government audit reports expenditure levels of 75% for NACP I and 46% for the first four years of NACP II, while NACO reports expenditure levels in the region of 98%–99%. NACO, *National AIDS Control Programme: Response to the HIV Epidemic in India*; World Bank, "Implementation Completion," 20; CAG, "Union Government"; NACO, "Funds and Expenditure." The budget number for NACP IV comes from a NACO strategy document; I converted the total budget figure of ₹13,415 crore at a conversion rate of US$1 = ₹64 (a 2017 exchange rate). NACO, "National AIDS Control Programme Phase IV (2012–2017)," 15.

2. Johnston and Ainsworth, "Project Performance Assessment Report," 4; NACO, *National AIDS Prevention and Control Policy*, 7; NACO, *NACP III*, 10–11; NACO, "National AIDS Control Programme Phase IV (2012–2017)," 9.

APPENDIX 2. Detailed are the duration, budget, and main components for four phases of Kenyan AIDS policy from 2000 to 2019. SOURCE: National AIDS Control Council (NACC) documents, compiled by author.

PHASE	DURATION	BUDGET[1]	MAIN PRIORITIES/STRATEGIES[2]
KNASP I (Kenya National AIDS Strategic Plan I)	2000–2005	$160 million	• Prevention and advocacy • Treatment, continuum of care, and support • Mitigation of the social and economic impacts of AIDS • Monitoring, evaluation, and research • Management and coordination
KNASP II	2005/6–2009/10	$2.0 billion	• Preventing new infections • Improving quality of life of those infected or affected by HIV • Mitigating the social and economic impact of AIDS
KNASP III	2009/10–2012/13	$3.6 billion	• Cost-effective prevention, treatment, care, and support services, • Mainstreaming of HIV in key sectors through long-term programming • Targeted, community-based programs • Coordination of stakeholders within a nationally owned strategy and aligned results framework • Cross-cutting focus on most-at-risk populations, including sex workers

Kenya AIDS Strategic Framework (KASF)	2014/15–2018/19	$5.5 billion	• Reducing new HIV infections • Improving health outcomes and wellness of all people living with HIV • Using a human rights approach to facilitate access to services for people living with HIV/AIDS, key populations, and other priority groups in all sectors • Strengthening integration of health and community systems • Strengthening research and innovation to inform KASF goals • Promoting utilization of strategic information for research and monitoring and evaluation to enhance programming • Increasing domestic financing for a sustainable HIV response • Promoting accountable leadership for delivery of the KASF results by all sectors and actors

1. For KNASP I, the budget amount is from the National AIDS Control Council (NACC). NACC reported a requirement of KSh14.059 billion (Kenya shillings), or US$160 million (year 2000), and an expected funding base of KSh7.735 billion, or US$88 million (year 2000). KNASP II reported a need for KSh179.452 billion, or US$2.0 billion (year 2005). KNASP III reported a need for KSh266.708 billion, or US$3.56 billion at a conversion of US$ = KSh75. KASF reported a need for US$5.4864 billion. All budget numbers are cost estimates of required funding, not actually available funding amounts (for example, in KNASP III, NACC reports that it has available only $2.5 billion of its $3.6 billion requirement). NACC, *Strategic Plan 2000–2005*, 19; NACC, *Strategic Plan 2005/6–2009/10*, 35; NACC, *Strategic Plan 2009/10–2012/13*, 35, 37; and NACC, "Kenya AIDS Strategic Framework," 50.
2. NACC, *Strategic Plan 2000–2005*, 4; NACC, *Strategic Plan 2005/6–2009/10*, vii; NACC, *Strategic Plan 2009/10–2012/13*, xiii; and NACC, "Kenya AIDS Strategic Framework," xi.

This book draws on a total of 153 in-depth interviews. Most were conducted between July 2012 and November 2013, but I continued conducting new interviews until 2015. In addition to these 153 interviews, I conducted 15 follow-up interviews in 2015 and 2017. Of the interview participants, 102 were sex workers and others targeted by HIV prevention programs, including cisgender women in sex work (52 in India, 16 in Kenya), gay and bisexual men and kothis (15 in India and five in Kenya), and transgender women (14 in India). These interviewees participated in HIV prevention as members, peer educators or supervisors, outreach workers, program managers, and elected leaders. In India, these interviews were spread across three organizations or groups of organizations, with multiple offices, all in Bangalore, and I conducted the interviews in Kannada. In Kenya, they were spread across two organizations, one in Nairobi and one in Mombasa. I conducted these interviews in English, or, in some cases, with the help of a translator in Swahili or Gikuyu.

In addition to these interviews, I conducted 50 interviews with organizational directors, state officials, donor representatives, researchers, lawyers, and allied activists, including from the labor, feminist, and Dalit movements. These interviewees were spread across a more varied geographic terrain; they were based in Delhi, Chennai, Kolkata, Sangli (Maharashtra), Bijapur

(Karnataka), and Pariyaram (Kerala) in India; in Nairobi and Mombasa in Kenya; and in Manitoba and New York in North America. These interviewees included two former directors of the National AIDS Control Organization and nationally and globally prominent activists. I also spoke informally with dozens of other experts and activists, including several in Durban and Cape Town in South Africa. My average interview was about an hour long, ranging from about half an hour to two and a half hours in length. Most of the interviews took place in organizational offices, which I quickly found to be the safest and most comfortable place for interviewees to speak with me. Of my 82 interviews in Kannada, I transcribed most (55) of the interviews myself directly into English from Kannada and hired three transcribers fluent in Kannada and English to transcribe the remaining 27 interviews. Of these, half (13) were then retranscribed or thoroughly checked by either me or another of the transcribers. I transcribed all 71 interviews I conducted in English myself.

My textual analysis included academic articles from the public health literature; NGO, government, and donor reports, including national- and state-level policy and training documents; websites; and, to map debates over India's AIDS crisis, 135 medical journal articles from 1985 to 1995 with a subset of about 50 opinion and review articles. I also reviewed about 50 newspaper articles published in the *Times of India* and the *New York Times*.

Between 2012 and 2017, my fieldwork included about 15 months in Bangalore (12 continuous months from 2012 to 2013 and then summer visits in 2015 and 2017) and three months in Nairobi, with trips to Kolkata, Delhi, Chennai, Sangli, Bijapur, Mysore, and Mombasa. During these trips, I typically visited an organization associated with the AIDS response I had met through a contact, interviewed key leaders, and spent time sitting in on meetings, having informal group discussions, and visiting project sites. In Kolkata, where I visited twice, I met with interviewees from a broader range of organizations and affiliations.

My fieldwork in Bangalore forms the bulk of the participant observation for this book. I hung out in drop-in centers and attended protests and public events. Once I built stronger relationships, I was invited to meetings, ran into people I knew on the bus, and visited homes. Where I was asked to do so, I was involved in organizational activities. These activities included things like designing and facilitating training on the legal context for sex work, editing a funding application, drafting a concept note for a research project, analyzing focus group data, and organizing voting at two different organizational elections. I even ended up giving a speech at an annual day event. I wrote fieldnotes every day and consolidated them into fieldwork memos every few months. Though a leader from one organization asked me to discontinue contact after 2015, I stayed in close touch with others for many years after. People I met during fieldwork have become friends, travel companions, and intellectual collaborators.

My initial access to my interlocutors emerged through a combination of prior contacts and out-of-the-blue emails, but mostly the latter. I was lucky. Several activists and organizational leaders I initially emailed put me in touch with long lists of colleagues for me to interview. As I triangulated documents, ethnographic fieldwork, and interviews, I gained a sense of key figures in the activist milieus I was studying, as well as the range of political articulations I wanted to chart. Attending the Sex Workers Freedom Festival in 2012 helped me map out sex worker activism in India. The bulk of my interviews, however, emerged through fieldwork in community organizations. The Committee for the Protection of Human Subjects at University of California, Berkeley, which approved my research protocol, required that I sign an agreement with organizations at which I intended to conduct a series of interviews and spend time engaged in participant observation. After that, I visited community organizations and asked people I met if I could interview them and then asked them for further contacts. In some cases, I was introduced to an interviewee by a program manager, but the candid and critical accounts that my interviewees shared suggest that these introductions did not necessarily predispose the narrative.

Nevertheless, a major challenge of research was moving past what sometimes felt like a rehearsed life story that many of my interviewees had often been called on to perform for researchers, donors, and foreign visitors. These limitations were an inherent feature of my research context, but I mitigated them to some degree with longer interviews; an open-ended interview guide with a very short list of demographic questions I asked only at the end; and, most importantly, spending enough time hanging around that, with many interviewees, I had multiple conversations and built a relationship over time. I was never the only researcher or student to pass through these transnationally connected places. But I did stick around for longer than most researchers conducting an evaluation or quick focus group, and I believe that helped me to gain a more nuanced picture of the intersection of HIV prevention and everyday life. As an Indian American, dominant-caste, US educated, English-speaking young woman, I was often initially perceived as an intern, or sometimes as a donor or public health researcher. My background inevitably affected the data I collected. Often, conversations about my own trajectory spurred conversations about marriage, caste, higher education, gender, and sexuality.

Clothing was a telling indicator of my negotiations of the spaces of HIV prevention. In a donor office, I might wear Western clothes and introduce myself with my best American twang; in a government office, I dressed with an eye to modesty and Indian middle-class respectability, speaking in more measured English; at a protest, I dressed a bit more casually and comfortably and spoke mainly in Kannada. This kind of code-switching and boundary-crossing was less dissimulation and more a product of my privilege and diasporic habitus. It will also be familiar to anyone who has navigated state institutions in South Asia as a feminine-presenting or gender- nonconforming person. The threat of sexual violence was ever present and shaped my navigations of public spaces in overt and subtle ways. Nevertheless, moving across a hybrid transnational terrain requires hybrid transnational strategies that my background and privilege equipped me uniquely to take on. It also meant I was often at risk of questioning, as when someone at a protest asked me if I was "really from America" or "just saying that," or when an organizational advisor accused me of secretly working for the Gates Foundation, or when Kenyan peer educators assumed I was another trainer or evaluator from India. These moments of presumed disloyalty reflect, in part, the contested terrain of HIV prevention, within which conflicting actors engaged in close proximity.

Notes

PREFACE

1. In this book, I follow UNAIDS guidelines in not using the term *HIV/AIDS*. I refer to *AIDS* when discussing the global pandemic and to *HIV* when discussing measures to prevent viral transmission. UNAIDS, *Terminology Guidelines*, 8.

2. Shahani, "How to Survive."

3. UNAIDS, *2006 Report on the Global AIDS Epidemic*, 374.

4. UNAIDS, "South Africa." In South Africa today, an estimated 7.5 million people are living with HIV.

5. UNAIDS and WHO, "AIDS Epidemic Update," 23.

6. Wines, "Durban Journal."

7. Klugman, "Politics of Contraception"; and Marks, "Epidemic Waiting to Happen?"

8. Lurie et al., "Impact of Migration"; Hunter, *Love in the Time of AIDS*; and Decoteau, *Ancestors and Antiretrovirals*.

9. Hunter, "Materiality of Everyday Sex."

10. Farmer, *AIDS and Accusation*; Comaroff, "Beyond Bare Life"; and Watkins-Hayes, "Intersectionality and the Sociology of HIV/AIDS."

11. Bishnupriya Ghosh, in "The Costs of Living," clarifies that female sex workers were the initial focus of HIV prevention programs in India; men who have sex with men became a focus somewhat later; and IV drug users were considered a less significant population, except in Northeastern India.

12. In this book, I use pseudonyms for everyone except for those it would be impossible to anonymize. For these people, I mostly rely on existing public

statements and documents or obtained their consent to identify them by name. While those familiar with the contexts I write about may be able to connect data with specific organizations, I have worked to ensure that it cannot be linked to specific people. Where details seem vague or jumbled, I have rendered them so deliberately, in order to maintain confidentiality to the furthest extent possible.

13. *Dalit*, meaning oppressed or crushed, is a term used to refer to groups formerly designated untouchable in the Indian caste system. The term *Dalit* emphasizes the systematic oppression of these groups; the census categorizes them as scheduled caste (SC) or scheduled tribe (ST).

14. PFI et al., *HIV/AIDS in Karnataka*, 20.

15. *High prevalence* indicated HIV prevalence higher than 1%.

16. PFI et al., *HIV/AIDS in Karnataka*, 6.

17. PFI et al., 9.

18. Following UNAIDS guidelines, I use the term sexually transmitted infection (STI). However, when a source uses an older term, such as venereal disease or sexually transmitted disease, I follow the terminology of the source. UNAIDS, *Terminology Guidelines*, 11.

19. *Kothi* is a vernacular term for a feminine man or gender-nonconforming person who prefers sex in the receptive role with other men. The term also often carries class connotations; it can refer to a working-class person in contrast to elite, English-speaking gay men. The term has a complex history. See L. Cohen, "Kothi Wars."

20. KSAPS, *Annual Action Plan 2012–2013*, 27.

21. Moses et al., "Intensive HIV Prevention"; and UNAIDS, *Global Report, 2010*, 34.

22. Ng et al., "Assessment of Population-Level Effect," 1649.

23. The UN's sixth Millennium Development Goal (MDG), set in 2000 to be met by 2015, committed member countries to "combat HIV/AIDS, malaria, and other diseases," which included the target of halting and reversing the spread of AIDS and achieving universal access to AIDS treatment.

24. UNAIDS, "India Overview."

CHAPTER 1: INTRODUCTION

Epigraph is from Rubin, "Thinking Sex, "267.

1. See Farmer, *AIDS and Accusation*; Farmer, *Infections and Inequalities*; Padilla, *Caribbean Pleasure Industry*; Mojola, *Love, Money, and HIV*; Wyrod, *AIDS and Masculinity*; Carrillo, *The Night Is Young*; Campbell, *Letting Them Die*, and Watkins-Hayes, "Intersectionality and the Sociology of HIV/AIDS."

2. See Blankenship et al., "Challenging the Stigmatization"; Alexander, *A Stranger Truth*; and Ng et al., "Assessment of Population-Level Effect."

3. See Epstein, *Impure Science*; Biehl, "Activist State"; Biehl, *Will to Live*; Gould, *Moving Politics*; Nguyen, *Republic of Therapy*; Decoteau, *Ancestors and Antiretrovirals*; Benton, *HIV Exceptionalism*; and Swidler and Watkins, *Fraught Embrace*.

4. Khanna, "Taming of the Shrewd Meyeli Chhele"; Boyce, "Conceiving 'Kothis'"; L. Cohen, "Kothi Wars"; Karnik, "Locating HIV/AIDS and India"; khanna, *Sexualness*; A. Dutta, "Legible Identities and Legitimate Citizens"; S. Ghosh, "Surveillance in Decolonized Social Space"; Chacko, *Chasing Numbers Betraying People*; ABVA, *Women and AIDS*; and ABVA, *Less Than Gay*.

5. Theories of biological citizenship often overlook the role of the state in delivering HIV care and in being a site of allegiance and aspiration. Benton, *HIV Exceptionalism*, 136.

6. Mahajan, "Philanthropy and the Nation-State."

7. I use the term *sex worker* to refer to people who exchange sex for money, though I recognize the term is shorthand and includes many who may not identify with this term. I use *sexual minority* as shorthand for accommodating a wide range of sexual identities, categories, and preferences, including gay, lesbian, bisexual, and *double-decker* (usually used to describe a masculine person who prefers both receptive and penetrative sex with men). My use of *transgender people* includes those who might call themselves *transgender*, as well as those who might call themselves *kothi* (usually used to describe an effeminate man or gender-nonconforming person who prefers receptive sex with men) or *hijra* (usually used to describe someone assigned masculine gender at birth who wears conventionally female clothing and participates in the hijra system of family relationships, religious and cultural traditions, and economic ties). I use these terms with the recognition that these terms are partial, shifting, and fluid, and that they often overlap. Nevertheless, I find these terms more broadly useful, and more aligned with the terms used by activists I foreground in this book, than the narrower epidemiological terms *female sex worker* and *men who have sex with men* that typically appear in public health literature.

8. Beck, *World at Risk*, 9.

9. Sangaramoorthy, "Treating the Numbers."

10. S. Mohan, "AIDS Scare in India."

11. See Casarett and Lantos, "Have We Treated AIDS Too Well?"; J. H. Smith and Whiteside, "History of AIDS Exceptionalism"; and Benton, *HIV Exceptionalism*.

12. NACO and ICMR, "India HIV Estimations," 21.

13. This figure comes from the OECD (Organisation for Economic Co-operation and Development) Creditor Reporting System (CRS). OECD countries report development aid to CRS annually, allowing for comparison across sectors. I compiled funding commitments from all donors for STD control, including HIV, to India between 1995 and 2018 in constant 2018 US dollars. STD control including HIV/AIDS does not fall under the health category in the CRS; it falls under population and reproductive health, of which it has constituted between 67% and 80% of official development assistance since 2003. The database includes both multilateral and bilateral donors and some private donors, but it does not account for domestic expenditure. I calculated the figure for commitments (not disbursements) for official development assistance for all channels and types of aid. The CRS also includes a category for social mitigation of HIV, which accounted for 2% of commitments under other social infrastructure and services in 2012.

14. UNAIDS, "India Overview." Accessed 2018. https://www.unaids.org/en/regionscountries/countries/india.

15. Dhingra et al., "Adult and Child Malaria," 4.

16. Jha et al., "HIV Mortality and Infection," 5.

17. These figures come from the OECD CRS. Here, I compiled data for official development assistance from all official donors (which includes bilateral, multilateral, and private aid) disbursed through all channels between 2002 and 2018 for STD control, including HIV, tuberculosis control, and malaria control. All figures are in constant 2017 US dollars.

18. This figure comes from the OECD CRS and refers to funding commitments to the categories of STD control, including HIV and health, total for all recipient countries, donors, types, and channels of aid, in constant 2018 US dollars.

19. In 2018, US$6.2 billion of worldwide official development assistance was committed to STD control, including HIV, compared to $10.9 billion in the entire health sector, according to my analysis of OECD CRS data.

20. UNAIDS, "Global HIV & AIDS Statistics: 2020 Fact Sheet."

21. Monika Krause writes in *The Good Project* about this field but focuses on humanitarian organizations, not states, as the unit of analysis.

22. Fourcade, "State Metrology."

23. De Souza's "Construction of HIV/AIDS in Indian Newspapers," covering the mid-2000s, notes the "nationalist" character of many accounts in which AIDS becomes "India's fight to be seen and acknowledged as a developed nation capable of managing its own problems independently and successfully" (p. 260).

24. Bourdieu and Wacquant, *Invitation to Reflexive Sociology*, 97.

25. Khanna, *Sexualness*, 77.

26. The field approach I use in this book differs from the idea of transnational governmentality that political anthropologists have developed. Take, for example, James Ferguson and Akhil Gupta's influential joint essay, "Spatializing States," in which they develop the concept of transnational governmentality. In an analysis of India and what they call "weak African states," they argue for the importance of understanding the spatial elements of state authority. In India, they show, metaphors of verticality and encompassment buttress the state's claim to authority: "higher up" officials are responsible for larger spatial areas. In Africa, they suggest that transnational agencies, not governments, play an active role in local governance. The essay is explicitly not comparative. But a field approach offers a way to understand how these dynamics of state spatiality are actually produced in relation to each other. The Indian state operates in a different relationship to global institutions than the Kenyan state, but both operate within the same global field.

27. The scholarship on global fields suggests a variety of ways in which fields and actors can emerge. For example, humanitarian fields are global from the start, while other global fields might emerge from national fields. The actors in a global field could be defined as individuals, organizations, and nation-states. Here, because of the particular nature of the global AIDS field, I consider nation-states to be actors in a global field structured and mediated by global institutions—both global governance institutions like UNAIDS and the WHO and private institutions with global aspirations, such as the Gates Foundation. Rather than mapping the global AIDS field, my goal here is to show how participation in the global field intersects with regional and local politics. Go and Krause, "Fielding Transnationalism"; and Krause, *Good Project*.

28. Fourcade, "State Metrology."

29. Latour, *Science in Action*, 227.

30. Collins, *Black Sexual Politics*, 44.

31. Enloe, *Bananas, Beaches and Bases*; Rai, "Gendering Global Governance"; and Peterson, "Political Identities."

32. D. Cooper, "Engaged State."

33. Mitchell, "Society, Economy, and the State Effect."

34. Puri, *Sexual States*.

35. Heng, "Great Way to Fly"; Yuval-Davis, "Gender and Nation"; Kempadoo, *Sexing the Caribbean*, 3; and Kim-Puri, "Conceptualizing Gender-Sexuality-State-Nation."

36. Alexander, "Not Just (Any) Body."

37. Peterson, "Political Identities"; and Duggan, "Queering the State."

38. Levine, *Prostitution, Race, and Politics*; and Whitehead, "Bodies Clean and Unclean."

39. Bhaskaran, "Politics of Penetration."

40. Puri, *Sexual States*; Pandit, "Gendered Subaltern Sexuality"; Gopal, "Ruptures and Reproduction"; Bacchetta, "When the (Hindu) Nation Exiles Its Queers"; and Kapur, "Citizen and the Migrant."

41. ABVA, *Women and AIDS*, 14–15.

42. NACO, *Targeted Interventions*, 7.

43. Benton, *HIV Exceptionalism*.

44. E. McDonnell, "Patchwork Leviathan."

45. See S. Ghosh, "Surveillance in Decolonized Social Space"; A. Dutta, "Legible Identities and Legitimate Citizens"; and Boyce and khanna, "Rights and Representations."

46. Surya, "Failed Radical Possibilities."

47. Khanna, *Sexualness*, 71.

48. Katyal, *Doubleness of Sexuality*, 42.

49. Menon, "Sexuality, Caste, Governmentality," 91. See also John, "Intersectionality"; Roy, *New South Asian Feminisms*, 10–11; Shah, "Sex Workers' Rights"; Murthy and Seshu, *Business of Sex*; and Siddiqi, "Sexuality, Rights and Personhood."

50. Brown, "Finding the Man"; Rai, "Women and the State"; and Rajan, *Scandal of the State*.

51. Connell, "State, Gender, and Sexual Politics."

52. Sharma, "Crossbreeding Institutions, Breeding Struggle," 65.

53. Political anthropologists approaching the state ethnographically have largely focused on three avenues for theorizing the state: as a symbolic representation, as a site and tool of governance, and as a site of contestation (e.g., Hansen et al., *States of Imagination*.) We can see all three of these functions in the response to AIDS in India.

54. Paschel, *Becoming Black Political Subjects*; and Paschel, "Disaggregating the Racial State." See also Buchholz, "What Is a Global Field?" This approach to the alignment of national and global fields differs from that of Keck and Sikkink, who argue in *Activists beyond Borders* that local social movements use a boomerang effect, accessing global institutions to put pressure on their national states. Here, global institutions constitute a varied field that may or may not find points of alignment with local activism.

55. Fourcade, "State Metrology."

56. Morgan and Orloff, *Many Hands.*

57. Burawoy, "Manufacturing the Global," 157.

58. Burawoy, *Global Ethnography,* 4.

59. Peck and Theodore, "Follow the Policy"; Massey, *Space, Place, and Gender*; and Hart, *Disabling Globalization.*

60. Grewal, *Transnational America*; Grewal and Kaplan, *Scattered Hegemonies*; Mohanty, "Under Western Eyes"; Mohanty, "'Under Western Eyes' Revisited"; and Puar, *Terrorist Assemblages.*

61. Bhambra, "Comparative Historical Sociology"; Patil, "From Patriarchy to Intersectionality"; and Patil, "Heterosexual Matrix."

62. Johnston and Ainsworth, "Project Performance Assessment Report," 1.

63. Patton, *Inventing AIDS.*

64. Burton, *Africa in the Indian Imagination.*

65. Mathur, *Paper Tiger*; and Puri, *Sexual States.* See also Hull, *Government of Paper*; A. Gupta, *Red Tape*; and Ferguson and Gupta, "Spatializing States."

66. Paschel, *Becoming Black Political Subjects, 242.*

67. Lakkimsetti, *Legalizing Sex*; khanna, *Sexualness*; and Puri, *Sexual States.*

68. B. Ghosh, "Costs of Living"; S. Mohan, *Towards Gender Inclusivity.*

69. But, see Chorev, *Give and Take.*

70. De Souza, "Construction of HIV/AIDS in Indian Newspapers," 260.

71. A. Ghosh, "World AIDS Day"; *India Today*, "India's AIDS Control Mission"; and NACO, "National AIDS Control Programme IV."

72. Cheng, Juhasz, and Shahani, *AIDS and the Distribution of Crises.* See also the concept of *syndemics*, which focuses on the interconnectedness of social and medical epidemics. Singer, *Introduction to Syndemics*; and Watkins-Hayes, *Remaking a Life.*

73. Berlant, "Slow Death (Sovereignty, Obesity, Lateral Agency)," 102.

74. S. Mohan, *Towards Gender Inclusivity,* 60.

75. Thompson et al., *Systematic Approach,* 45.

76. Rau, *Avahan-India AIDS Initiative,* 7–8.

77. Steinmetz, "Octopus and the Hekatonkheire," 387.

78. Hart, *Disabling Globalization.*

79. Collins, *Black Sexual Politics.*

80. Viterna, *Women in War*; and Berry, *War, Women, and Power.*

81. Hall, "Cultural Studies and Its Theoretical Legacies," 271.

82. Hall, *Cultural Studies 1983*; and Vijayakumar, "Sexual Laborers and Entrepreneurial Women."

83. Vijayakumar, "Sexual Laborers and Entrepreneurial Women."

84. F. L. Smith, *Sex and the Citizen*, 11; and Alexander, "Not Just (Any) Body," 15.

CHAPTER 2: INDIA AND THE SPECTER OF AFRICAN AIDS

1. G. P. Dutta, "Problems of AIDS," 254.

2. G. P. Dutta, 255.

3. Mehra, "Problems of AIDS."

4. Lal and Mertens, "HIV and AIDS," 77.

5. Jayaraman, "AIDS in Position to Ravage India."

6. Farmer, *AIDS and Accusation*.

7. Treichler, "AIDS, Homophobia and Biomedical Discourse"; Sontag, *AIDS and Its Metaphors*; and Farmer, *AIDS and Accusation*.

8. Notably, this frequent invocation of the "African" epidemic masked considerable variation in the characteristics of the epidemic in different African countries. Patton, "Inventing 'African AIDS.'"

9. See Mahajan, "Designing Epidemics," for a discussion of how foreknowledge from African epidemics shaped Indian estimates of the future of HIV.

10. This chapter builds on fascinating textual studies of media representations of AIDS in India. All three studies note the contrasts between India and the West that shape postcolonial preoccupations about AIDS and Indian sexuality in mainstream US media in 2008, in English-language Indian media in 2004–2005, and in the global medical literature in the early 1980s.

11. Patton, "Inventing 'African AIDS,'" 37.

12. Benton, *HIV Exceptionalism*, 119.

13. Burton, *Africa in the Indian Imagination*; Khubchandani, "Voguing in Bangalore"; and Radhakrishnan, "Time to Show Our True Colors."

14. Though I use the term *sex worker* throughout the book, I use the term *prostitute* when it is the term used in my sources. The term *sex work* was not in use until the 1970s. Leigh, "Inventing Sex Work."

15. Krause, *Good Project*. See also Peck and Theodore, "Mobilizing Policy," for a discussion of fields of transnational expertise.

16. Krause, *Good Project*, 5.

17. Harris, *Achieving Access*.

18. Kang, "India May Face an Africa-like AIDS Situation."

19. Steinmetz, "Colonial State as a Social Field"; Steinmetz, "Octopus and the Hekatonkheire"; Go, "Global Fields and Imperial Forms"; and Go, *Postcolonial Thought and Social Theory*.

20. Kothari, "Authority and Expertise"; Hodge, "British Colonial Expertise"; and F. Cooper, "Writing the History."

21. In this book, I use the terms *prostitution, prostitute, female prostitute*, and *women in prostitution* when referring to historical time periods and contemporary institutional contexts in which these terms are the ones most often used. In all other contexts, I use the terms *sex work* and *sex worker*.

22. Levine, *Prostitution, Race, and Politics*, 2.

23. Legg, *Prostitution and the Ends of Empire*.

24. Nair, "Devadasi, Dharma and the State"; Vijaisri, "Contending Identities"; Tambe, *Codes of Misconduct*; and Ramberg, "When the Devi Is Your Husband."

25. Ramberg, "Magical Hair as Dirt"; Levine, "Venereal Disease"; Levine, *Prostitution, Race, and Politics*; Levine, "Multitude of Unchaste Women"; Whitehead, "Bodies Clean and Unclean"; and Tambe, *Codes of Misconduct*.

26. Tambe, "Elusive Ingénue"; and White, *Comforts of Home*.

27. Levine, "Rereading the 1890s."

28. Burton, *Burdens of History*.

29. Andrew and Bushnell, *Queen's Daughters in India*, 22, 34.

30. Levine, *Prostitution, Race, and Politics*, 292.

31. Bhaskaran, "Politics of Penetration."

32. Arondekar, *For the Record, Mitra, Indian Sex Life*.

33. Levine, *Prostitution, Race, and Politics*.

34. Burton, *Burdens of History*; and R. Gupta, "In Kolkata." See also Doezema, "Ouch!"

35. *Times of India*, "AIDS Vaccine Not a Breakthrough Yet."

36. *Times of India*, "WHO to Set up AIDS Panel."

37. *Times of India*, "Blood Transfusion Test for AIDS"; and *Times of India*, "Don't Import AIDS via Blood."

38. *Times of India*, "Indian Sex Taboos Ward off AIDS."

39. S. Sen, "West Bengal Guards against AIDS."

40. Ghosh, "AIDS."

41. Khurana, "AIDS."

42. Dube, *Sex, Lies and AIDS*, 1.

43. L. Cohen, "Song for Pushkin."

44. Catherine Yuk-Ping Lo, for example, notes that in China, early representations of AIDS translated to "love capitalism disease." Cheng, Juhasz, and Shahani, *AIDS and the Distribution of Crises*, 47.

45. *Times of India*, "Russia Untouched by AIDS."

46. Jayaraman, "India against AIDS."

47. *Times of India,* "India's First AIDS Clinic at J.J."

48. *Times of India,* "AIDS Centre for Madras Hospital."

49. Padabidri, "AIDS Threat."

50. Parakal, "AIDS Threat." Parakal was a veteran writer of letters to the editor and had some five thousand letters to the editor published between 1954 and 2005, one thousand of them in the *Times of India.* Aranha, "Mightier Than the Sword."

51. *Times of India,* "AIDS Centre for Madras Hospital."

52. *Times of India,* "AIDS Will Spread to Heterosexuals"; and "Current Topics."

53. Malik, "Way Fatal AIDS Disease Spreads."

54. *Times of India,* "Who's to Be Blamed for AIDS?"; Malik, "Way Fatal AIDS Disease Spreads."

55. *Times of India,* "Doctor Warns of AIDS Epidemic."

56. T. J. John et al., "Prevalence of HIV Infection."

57. *New York Times,* "71 AIDS Cases."

58. These broad generalizations, of course, obscured the fact that heterosexual women, particularly of color, in the US and homosexual men in many African countries were facing a devastating AIDS epidemic, largely overlooked by medical institutions until the 2000s.

59. If 2.9% of the seventy homosexual men tested had been seropositive, the same percentage as in the female prostitutes, they would have found two HIV-positive cases.

60. Asthana, "AIDS-Related Policies, Legislation and Programme Implementation," 186.

61. Jayaraman, "Pool of Infected Women?"

62. Jayaraman, "India Screens Foreign Students." These two groups were sometimes conflated. For example, a March 1987 article in *Nature* reported, "Indian health officials say that AIDS reached India chiefly through tourists and foreign students. Of the 104 cases so far identified, 11 were foreign students, 11 were tourists and 76 were female prostitutes; only five were Indian males." The prostitutes, the article continued, "claim to have had sexual relations with foreign priests attending Christian conventions." Presumably, the 76 female prostitutes were Indian but AIDS was mainly a problem of "tourists and foreign students." Jayaraman, "AIDS Institute for India?"

63. Jayaraman, "India Screens Foreign Students." A 1987 article suggests a more specific figure, that "more than 80 percent" of foreign students in India were African, but no source is cited for the figure. Jayaraman, "Students in India Object."

64. T. J. John et al., "Prevalence of HIV Infection," 160.

65. Jayaraman, "India Screens Foreign Students."

66. Jayaraman, "Students in India Object."

67. *New York Times*, "Africa Student."

68. Jayaraman, "AIDS Institute for India?"

69. HIV testing was required of visa applicants planning to spend more than a year in India.

70. Jayaraman, "Drastic Measures Proposed in India"; Hazarika, "To Fight AIDS"; and Bhargava and Devadas, "People Say There Is a Lot of Sex."

71. Songok et al., "Passage to India"; and Human Rights Watch, "India: Confirm Policy Ending Mandatory HIV Tests." Though a circular to this effect was issued in 2002, the expectations remained unclear until 2010, when the Ministry of External Affairs issued a fresh statement. Roy, "India to Its Missions: Don't Ask for Tests of Visa Applicants."

72. ABVA, *Women and AIDS*, 20; and Inderjit, "Even Hospitals Reject AIDS Patients."

73. In her influential piece "Dalit Women Talk Differently" (WS-43), for example, Sharmila Rege points to the "rounding up of prostitutes and segregating those found to be HIV positive" as part of the project of brahminical Hindutva to use gender issues as a site for cultural assertion against the West. See also Bacchetta, "When the (Hindu) Nation Exiles Its Queers."

74. Mahajan, "Designing Epidemics."

75. James Chin was chief of surveillance at the Global Programme on AIDS at the WHO. Chin's projections in 1990 used Delphi projections—in which fourteen "experts" were systematically asked to estimate the progress of the epidemic—to predict that the number of people worldwide living with HIV by 2000, without coordinated intervention programs, could reach over 18 million. The projections classified Asia, the Pacific, and North Africa as Pattern III countries. (Pattern I was Australia, New Zealand, western Europe, and the Americas, and Pattern II was sub-Saharan Africa and parts of the Caribbean.) The authors' projections suggested that the "largest relative increase in HIV prevalence (13-fold) is expected in areas currently classified as Pattern III." More specifically, the authors argued that "Asia may expect a tenfold increase in AIDS cases by the end of 1991 because the AIDS epidemic in most Asian countries is still at a very early stage when the doubling time for AIDS cases is much shorter than it will be later in the epidemic—a phenomenon already observed in Africa and the Americas." Chin, Sato, and Mann, "Projections of HIV Infections." Notably, in 2006, Chin published a book arguing that these kinds of predictions were overblown. Chin and Gillies, *AIDS Pandemic.*

76. Dube, *Sex, Lies and AIDS*, 115.

77. Jayaraman, "Disaster Looms for Bombay."

78. *Lancet*, "India."

79. Tanne, "AIDS Spreads Eastward."

80. Hazarika, "In an Unaware India."

81. Mangla, "India," 1534.

82. *Times of India*. "Coming to the AIDS of Asia."

83. Chowdhury, "AIDS Prevention," 304.

84. Chowdhury, 304.

85. Murmu, "AIDS."

86. Chitre, "AIDS Mania." Some of this skepticism took unusual forms. A letter to the editor in 1994 complained that activists who had portrayed the AIDS virus as a dinosaur were "misinformed about the creature" and noted, "Dinosaurs had never spread any disease whatsoever, let alone AIDS which is caused due to perverse sex—a purely human misadventure." *Times of India* "AIDS and Dinosaurs."

87. Mangla, "India," 1533.

88. Murmu, "AIDS."

89. Jayaraman and Macilwain, "India Moves Ahead Cautiously."

90. Imam, "India's AIDS Control Programme."

91. *AIDS Weekly*, "WHO Says Indian AIDS Funds Misused," 7–8.

92. Mehta, "400 Million Condoms."

93. Mehta.

94. Jayaraman, "AIDS in Position to Ravage India."

95. Shreedhar, "Dallying with Death," 16.

96. Imam, "India's AIDS Control Programme"; and Padki, "Controlling AIDS." In 1999, I. S. Gilada was arrested on charges of providing a false vaccine to a patient who later died. He was acquitted in 2009. Gilada's website credits him as "the first person to raise the alarm against AIDS in India" and a "globally acclaimed HIV expert, credited with bringing India on the AIDS control map of the world." Gilada, response to "Doctor in India arrested"; and Virology Education, "Ishwar Gilada, MD, DDV, FCPS."

97. World Bank, "Implementation Completion," 7.

98. Brookmeyer et al., "AIDS Epidemic in India."

99. Bollinger, Tripathy, and Quinn, "Human Immunodeficiency Virus Epidemic," 103–4. See also Bartlett, "AIDS in India"; and Pais, "HIV and India."

100. Jayaraman, "AIDS in Position to Ravage India."

101. Pais, "HIV and India."

102. *AIDS Weekly Plus*, "India AIDS Situation." See also Varam, "AIDS Situation Explosive."

103. Altman, "India Suddenly Leads in H.I.V."

104. UNAIDS and WHO, *Report on the Global HIV/AIDS Epidemic June 1998*, 13.

105. Burns, "Denial and Taboo Blinding India."

106. Eberstadt, "Future of AIDS," 22. See also National Intelligence Council, "Next Wave of HIV/AIDS"; and O'Manique, "Global Neoliberalism and AIDS Policy."

107. Dalal, "AIDS Bomb."

108. Antia, "AIDS Scare," Letters.

109. Priya, "AIDS, Public Health, and the Panic Reaction."

110. Mohan, "AIDS Scare in India." NACO, *National AIDS Control Programme: Response to the HIV Epidemic in India*.

111. Mahajan, "Designing Epidemics."

112. Booth, *Local Women, Global Science*; Kreiss et al., "AIDS Virus Infection"; and D'Costa et al., "Prostitutes Are a Major Reservoir."

113. Kreiss et al., "AIDS Virus Infection."

114. Kreiss et al., "AIDS Virus Infection"; and D'Costa et al., "Prostitutes Are a Major Reservoir."

115. White, *Comforts of Home*.

116. D'Costa et al., "Prostitutes Are a Major Reservoir," 64.

117. In South Africa, this model, which assumed that male migrants acquired HIV from sex workers and then spread HIV to their stationary female partners in rural areas, represented a new application of earlier models of the spread of syphilis under apartheid migrant labor systems. Booth, *Local Women, Global Science*; and Hunter, "Beyond the Male-Migrant."

118. Mitra, *Indian Sex Life*.

119. UNAIDS, *2006 Report on the Global AIDS Epidemic*, 511.

120. Dandona et al., "Is the HIV Burden in India Being Overestimated?"

121. UNAIDS, *Report on the Global HIV/AIDS Epidemic 2008*, 219.

122. UNAIDS, "2.5 Million People"; and McNeil, "India, Said to Play Down AIDS."

123. Dandona et al., "Sex Behaviour."

124. See ABVA, *Less Than Gay*.

125. C. Cohen, *Boundaries of Blackness*; Watkins-Hayes, "Intersectionality and the Sociology of HIV/AIDS"; and Watkins-Hayes, *Remaking a Life*.

126. Schulman, *Gentrification of the Mind*; and Shahani, "How to Survive."

127. Paschel, "Disaggregating the Racial State."

CHAPTER 3: FROM CONTAINMENT TO INCORPORATION

1. Evans, *Embedded Autonomy*. See also Harris, *Achieving Access*, on elite advocacy in global health.

2. Evans and Heller, "State and Development," 121.

3. Ray and Katzenstein, *Social Movements in India*; and Kudva, "Strong States, Strong NGOs."

4. E. McDonnell, "Patchwork Leviathan."

5. Paschel, *Becoming Black Political Subjects*.

6. Roychowdhury, *Capable Women, Incapable States*; and Sharma, *Logics of Empowerment*.

7. See Amar, *Security Archipelago*, for an account of shifting logics of sexual governance.

8. This process parallels work by scholars who show how, rather than transforming patriarchal, racist, and heteronormative practices at large, state agencies incorporate Black, feminist, or sex worker activists into some parts of the state. Sharma, *Logics of Empowerment*; Paschel, "Disaggregating the Racial State"; and Rivers-Moore, "Waiting for the State."

9. E. McDonnell, "Patchwork Leviathan."

10. Misra, "Politico-Moral Transactions."

11. Tambe, *Codes of Misconduct*.

12. *Prostitution, Race, and Politics*, 63.

13. Hodges, "'Looting' the Lock Hospital," 391.

14. Levine, *Prostitution, Race, and Politics*, 92.

15. Legg, *Prostitution and the Ends of Empire*.

16. Tambe, *Codes of Misconduct*.

17. Debates crystallized around the *dēvadāsi* system, a courtesan tradition that officials increasingly conflated with prostitution. In 1909, the Mysore princely state abolished the dēvadāsi system, and in 1934 and 1947, Bombay and Madras followed suit. Ramberg, *Given to the Goddess*; Kannabiran, "Judiciary, Social Reform and Debate"; Sixty-Fourth Report on the Suppression of Immoral Traffic in Women and Girls Act, 1956, Law Commission of India, Act 104 of 1956, Parliament (1975); Nair, "Devadasi, Dharma and the State"; and Vijaisri, "Contending Identities."

18. These laws formed the basis of the postindependence Suppression of Immoral Traffic Act, which in turn formed the basis of the Immoral Traffic (Prevention) Act in force today.

19. Tambe, *Codes of Misconduct*; and Legg, *Prostitution and the Ends of Empire*.

20. Asthana, "AIDS-Related Policies, Legislation and Programme Implementation in India."

21. Dube, *Indefinite Sentence*, 124.

22. Jayaraman, "Pool of Infected Women?"

23. *Lancet*, "India."

24. *Lancet*, "India."

25. ABVA, *Women and AIDS*, 47–48.

26. Dube, *Indefinite Sentence*, 205.

27. See also Chapter 9 of ABVA, *Less Than Gay*.

28. ABVA, *Women and AIDS*, 38.

29. ABVA, 40.

30. SIAAP, "SIAAP Story"; and Nataraj, "Indian Prostitutes." I have used the number mentioned in interviews.

31. Misra, "Politico-Moral Transactions," 47.

32. UNAIDS guidelines, for example, now stipulate the use of the term *key populations* instead of *high-risk groups* "in the sense of being key to the epidemic's dynamics or key to the response." This shift reflects a broader trend in the literature on HIV and AIDS toward less stigmatizing language. Notably, UNAIDS still distinguishes *key population* from *vulnerable populations*, "which are subject to societal pressures or social circumstances that may make them more vulnerable to exposure to infections, including HIV." The distinction separates the more stigmatized groups at risk of HIV from, for example, orphans, who are part of the *vulnerable* category, and hints at a continued assumption that some populations are more innocent and less responsible for HIV risk than others. UNAIDS, *Terminology Guidelines*, 8. See also Dancy-Scott et al., "Trends in HIV Terminology."

33. Johnston and Ainsworth, "Project Performance Assessment Report," 41.

34. As interviewees explained to me, NACO was headed by a high-ranking official at the secretary level rather than a more junior deputy director general, as with other disease control programs.

35. Kadri and Kumar, "Institutionalization of the NACP."

36. Indian HIV prevention programs would later evolve in a distinct direction. See, for example, SANGRAM's critique of the 100% Condom Programme. Center for Advocacy on Stigma and Marginalisation, *Rights-Based Sex Worker Empowerment Guidelines*.

37. NACO, *National AIDS Control Policy*, 22.

38. Human Rights Watch, *Epidemic of Abuse*, 14–15. See also Lakkimsetti, *Legalizing Sex*.

39. Human Rights Watch, *Epidemic of Abuse*, 22.

40. Human Rights Watch, 12,19.

41. Human Rights Watch, 28.

42. Decoteau, "Exclusionary Inclusion."

43. NACO, *Targeted Interventions*, 16.

44. NACO, 27.

45. NACO, 16.

46. NACO, 141.

47. Compared to later donors, the World Bank generally downplayed its role. A Bank document from the time notes that "a more public advocacy role by the Bank . . . could have strengthened the perception that the HIV/AIDS program was externally driven." Johnston and Ainsworth, "Project Performance Assessment Report," 11.

48. G. Mohan and Stokke, "Participatory Development and Empowerment"; and Escobar, "Place, Nature and Culture."

49. Johnston and Ainsworth, "Project Performance Assessment Report," ix.

50. NACO, *National AIDS Control Programme: Response to the HIV Epidemic in India*, 13.

51. There was often more money than the government could spend. A 2003 government audit argued that "NACO should immediately assess the unspent balances lying with the State AIDS cells," as some "could not utilize even 25 per cent of the funds provided to them." Both NACP I and NACP II were extended by two years each when they were unable to absorb funds, which a World Bank evaluation explained as the result of both low capacity and the availability of extensive additional funds. World Bank, "Implementation Completion," 9, 20; and CAG, "Union Government."

52. Ng et al., "Assessment of Population-Level Effect," 1643.

53. Data on official development assistance come from the OECD CRS and are in constant 2018 US dollars. For foreign contribution data, I compiled funding amounts for HIV/AIDS from the Foreign Contribution Regulation Act (FCRA) annual reports between 2005 and 2012. At the peak of foreign contributions for HIV/AIDS, in 2008–2009, they comprised ₹1,049 crore, or about US$175 million in 2009 dollars. Between 2001 and 2007, foreign contributions for HIV/AIDS comprised between 0.5% and 4.2% of all foreign contributions; in 2011–2012 they comprised 2% of foreign contributions.

54. NACO, "Funds and Expenditure."

55. While high-risk groups technically included female sex workers, IV drug users, and men who have sex with men under the NACP, female sex workers tended to dominate the agenda and the public face of HIV prevention until the mid-2000s. At the end of NACP II, state AIDS control societies reported having reached just 6% of men who have sex with men through targeted interventions

compared to 35–45% of female sex workers. World Bank, "Implementation Completion," 34.

56. NACO, *National AIDS Control Policy*, 5.

57. NACO, *National AIDS Control Programme: Response to the HIV Epidemic in India*, 15.

58. NACO, 14.

59. NACO, *Targeted Interventions*, 15.

60. NACO, *National AIDS Control Programme Phase IV: Strategic Approach*, 32.

61. Kotiswaran, *Dangerous Sex, Invisible Labor.*

62. Lakkimsetti, "Governing Sexualities"; and Lakkimsetti, "HIV Is Our Friend."

63. Lawyer's Collective, "Statement from the National Consultation."

64. Armstrong and Bernstein, "Culture, Power, and Institutions," 93. In posing a *multi-institutional* alternative to dominant strands of political process theory, the authors point out that thinking about social movements as targeting multiple institutions beyond the state allows theorists to consider how social movements can exploit contradictions across institutions. Here, contradictions among institutions *within* the state created opportunities for social movements.

65. Dasgupta, "Of Raids and Returns"; VAMP, SANGRAM; and Rights4Change, *Raided.*

66. Kole, "Globalizing Queer?"

67. See Chatterjee, "AIDS in India." See also Rao, "How the LGBTQ Fight in India Went from Being a Health Issue to Civil Rights" for an account of how a visit with an NGO in Bangalore shaped the then NACO director's perspective on the fight against Section 377.

68. See also Jyoti Puri's account of these legal battles, *Sexual States*, in which she documents the critiques of the Naz Foundation in the early years of Section 377 protests by other LGBTQIA+ activists and points to the limits of the use of AIDS as justification for decriminalizing homosexuality.

69. For further discussion of these kinds of contestations in HIV prevention programs, see Vijayakumar, "Collective Demands and Secret Codes."

70. See also Nataraj, "Indian Prostitutes Highlight AIDS Dilemma."

71. Nataraj had been organizing with sex workers since the late 1980s.

72. BIRDS had worked in rural development in northern Karnataka since 1980 but received a grant from the Dutch human rights NGO Hivos to begin HIV prevention work in 1993.

73. DMSC, "Durbar Mahila Samanwaya Committee."

74. Jenkins, *Female Sex Worker HIV Prevention Projects*.

75. Jana et al., "Sonagachi Project," 406.

76. DMSC, "Sex Workers' Manifesto."

77. See S. Ghosh's "Elusive Choice and Agency" and *Gendered Proletariat* for analysis of the manifesto and its contradictions.

78. Gooptu and Bandyopadhyay, "Rights to Stop the Wrong."

79. See *Budhadev Karmaskar v. State of West Bengal*, 135 of 2010 (India Supreme Court 2011).

80. Point of View, *Of Veshyas, Vamps, Whores, and Women*.

81. SANGRAM, "About Us."

82. SANGRAM, "Collectives."

83. Sahni and Shankar, *First Pan-India Survey*.

84. VAMP, SANGRAM, and Rights4Change, *Raided*.

85. Center for Advocacy on Stigma and Marginalisation, *Rights-Based Sex Worker Empowerment Guidelines*.

86. Thomas, "Spotlight on Meena Seshu, SANGRAM."

87. Point of View, *Of Veshyas, Vamps, Whores, and Women*, 26–27.

88. Jenkins, *Female Sex Worker HIV Prevention Projects*, 11–12.

89. Jenkins, 86.

90. UNAIDS, *2006 Report on the Global AIDS Epidemic*, 109.

91. The anti-prostitution pledge, or anti-prostitution loyalty oath, was applied to US-based organizations as well as foreign-funded organizations. A 2013 Supreme Court case ruled that the requirement violated the First Amendment rights to free speech of private agencies in the US. A 2020 decision authored by Justice Kavanaugh ruled that the requirement was still relevant to foreign organizations, who, the court said, did not possess First Amendment rights. *United States Leadership against HIV/AIDS, Tuberculosis, and Malaria Act of 2003, H.R. 1298, 108th Cong. (2003-2004); Agency for International Development et al. v. Alliance for Open Society International, Inc., et al., 12 (US Supreme Court 2013); and Agency for International Development v. Alliance for Open Society International, Inc., et al., 19 (US Supreme Court 2020).*

92. Pai, "Of a Pledge and a People."

93. Ban Ki-Moon, "Address to the International AIDS Conference."

94. The 2007 *UNAIDS Guidance Note on HIV and Sex Work* emphasized reducing entry into sex work and promoting "access to decent work"—an idea antithetical to the labor argument for sex work that activist groups espoused.

95. UNAIDS, *UNAIDS Guidance Note on HIV and Sex Work*, 2012.

96. Verma, Seth, and Subramanium, "Report of the Committee"; and SANGRAM, "Submissions to Panels."

97. Lakkimsetti, *Legalizing Sex*, 92.

98. Aretxaga, "Maddening States."

99. See Sharma, "Crossbreeding Institutions, Breeding Struggle" for a discussion of how NGOs can take on and remove "state garb" in order to pursue different ends.

100. Aretxaga, "Maddening States."

101. Horton, "Police and the Policed," shows how encounters with police are a complex site of power and desire.

102. A. Gupta, "Blurred Boundaries."

103. Fuller and Harriss, "For an Anthropology."

104. Morgan and Orloff, *Many Hands*.

105. Sharma, *Logics of Empowerment*, xxii. See also Misra, "Politico-Moral Transactions."

CHAPTER 4: AT-RISK CITIZENS

1. *The Hindu*, "Pension Parishad."

2. In using the term *citizen*, I draw particularly on scholarship about how sexually marginalized people engage with and make demands on the state (e.g., Richardson, "Rethinking Sexual Citizenship").

3. I explore the uses of this term further in Vijayakumar, "Collective Demands and Secret Codes."

4. Hall, *Cultural Studies 1983*, 142.

5. Hall, 143.

6. Vijayakumar, "Sexual Laborers and Entrepreneurial Women."

7. Raka Ray's account of Calcutta's political culture and her comparison of Calcutta and Bombay, in *Fields of Protest*, is my starting point here. The Communist Party (Marxist) (CPM) stable hold on West Bengal politics was beginning to weaken just when DMSC was beginning to form its political agenda. In 2011, the TMC won a majority in the state assembly elections, effectively ending thirty-four years of CPM rule. Thus, starting in the late 1990s, Kolkata's political field was becoming less centralized but was still dominated by the language and history of workers' rights. DMSC's approach was thus infused with the ideological elements of left political culture and labor rhetoric without necessarily actively pursuing participation in party politics. See Bardhan et al., "Changing Voting Patterns."

8. Yengkhom, "Sex Worker Invited."

9. An interviewee from SANLAAP, a prominent organization that has worked with women and children in Sonagachi since the 1980s, who opposes the idea that sex work is work explained that SANLAAP's work in Sonagachi had been

reduced to a much smaller scale because "DMSC does not want us to work in the middle of Sonagachi."

10. Murthy and Seshu, *Business of Sex*, 36–37.

11. Ramberg, *Given to the Goddess*; and Murthy and Seshu, *Business of Sex*.

12. Friedman, "Bangalore." For more informed perspectives on the city, see Srinivas, *Landscapes of Urban Memory*; Nair, *Promise of the Metropolis*; and Inglis, *Narrow Fairways*.

13. Holt, "Global Cities."

14. Radhakrishnan, "Examining the 'Global' Indian Middle Class"; Radhakrishnan, *Appropriately Indian*; and Upadhya and Vasavi, *In an Outpost*.

15. Benjamin, "Governance, Economic Settings and Poverty"; and RoyChowdhury, "Bringing Class Back In."

16. I compiled these data from the Foreign Contribution Regulation Act (FCRA) annual reports from 2005 and 2012. Organizations in India are required to report their foreign contributions to the government under FCRA.

17. One interviewee directly traced this dynamic to the Mysore princely state, a modernizing welfare state. See Nair, *Mysore Modern*.

18. Nair, *Promise of the Metropolis*, 87, 307–13.

19. Kudva, "Uneasy Relations."

20. Mount, "Not a Hijra."

21. Queer nightlife scholar Kareem Khubchandani writes of Bangalore as "a regional urban haven for queer and transgender migrants on account of its urban and economic development and its sophisticated NGO/nonprofit complex," a place visitors from Bombay and Delhi deemed unsophisticated, but precisely for this reason, a rich site for studying the imbrication of changing economic conditions and queer life. Khubchandani, *Ishtyle*, 21–22. See also Khubchandani, "Staging Transgender Solidarities."

22. Humsafar Trust, "About Us."

23. Naz Foundation, "Story of Naz."

24. Sangama, "About Us."

25. Swabhava, "About."

26. In Bangalore, given its particular trajectory of economic growth, language politics are a potent index of class division and often a political flashpoint. Nair, *Promise of the Metropolis*, 234–270.

27. Hijras are part of a ritual community of transgender women with its own religious practices and kinship structure. Hijras have a history in South Asia dating back to at least the sixteenth century. See Reddy, *With Respect to*

Sex. Many of my interviewees who were transgender women had participated in the hijra community at some point, but some had left the community and no longer identified primarily as hijra.

28. PUCL-K, *Human Rights Violations,* 61.

29. PUCL-K, *Human Rights Violations,* 63.

30. PUCL-K, *Human Rights Violations.* See also PUCL-K, *Policing Morality in Channapatna;* and Narrain, "Articulation of Rights."

31. S. Mohan, *Towards Gender Inclusivity.*

32. Payana, "About Payana."

33. Alexander, *Stranger Truth,* 14.

34. Rau, *Avahan-India AIDS Initiative,* 10.

35. PFI et al., *HIV/AIDS in Karnataka,* 7.

36. Ng et al., "Assessment of Population-Level Effect."

37. Swasti, "Chapter 15"; and Euser et al., "Pragati."

38. Chacko, "Chasing Numbers Betraying People."

39. Vijayakumar, Chacko, and Panchanadeswaran, "As Human Beings"; PUCL-K, *Policing Morality in Channapatna.*

40. PUCL-K, *Policing Morality in Channapatna.*

41. In 2013–14, the organization formally registered as Sadhana Mahila Sangha.

42. Sheth, "Sex, Sex Workers, and the City."

43. Vimochana, "Open Letter."

44. See Atluri's "Prerogative of the Brave" for a more thorough, critical exploration of hijra clapping and sexual citizenship.

45. Setting out to work with this diverse set of members, with diverse relationships to sex work and sexual norms, was not without its tensions. See Vijayakumar, "Is Sex Work Sex or Is Sex Work Work?"

46. Puri, *Sexual States.*

47. This account recalls the importance of identity cards in informal workers' movements in India, as in Agarwala's *Informal Labor, Formal Politics.*

48. Altman, "Globalization, Political Economy, and HIV/AIDS"; Khan, "Culture, Sexualities, and Identities"; Karnik, "Locating HIV/AIDS and India"; khanna, "Taming of the Shrewd Meyeli Chhele"; S. Ghosh, "Surveillance in Decolonized Social Space"; and A. Dutta, "Legible Identities and Legitimate Citizens."

49. Patton, *Inventing AIDS.*

50. VHS, NACO, and KHPT, *Global Fund for AIDS,* 124.

51. VHS, NACO, and KHPT, 129.

CHAPTER 5: RISKY SELVES

1. Interestingly, Preethi saw her life in the hijra system as lacking exposure to the outside, when both hijras and sex workers often stand in as symbols for public space, the street, and the associated dangers and desires. Her idea of outside seemed to have particular classed connotations. See Phadke, Khan, and Ranade, *Why Loiter?*

2. In the formulation I heard most often, the sentence was in Kannada, but the words *rough* and *smooth* were in English.

3. See Altman, "Globalization, Political Economy, and HIV/AIDS"; and Karnik, "Locating HIV/AIDS and India."

4. L. Cohen, "Kothi Wars."

5. See KHPT, *Evaluation of Community Mobilization.*

6. Watkins-Hayes, *Remaking a Life.* See also Robins, "From 'Rights' to 'Ritual.'"

7. Mahmood, *Politics of Piety,* 166.

8. Balogun and Hoang, "Political Economy of Embodiment."

9. Sazana Jayadeva, in "Below English Line" (593), shows how, for aspiring middle-class English language learners in Bangalore, speaking English was about not only language but also a new way of existing, of clothing and behavior. These dynamics were clear to many of those I interviewed, who noted the middle-class habitus, including speaking in English, that they learned through NGO work.

10. Jocelyn Viterna, in "Pulled, Pushed, and Persuaded" and *Women in War,* offers an approach to identity-based mobilization that traces identities before mobilization and how they are reinforced and/or transformed during movement participation. Her approach informs the analysis here. Ann Swidler and Susan Watkins, in *Fraught Embrace,* also offer accounts of the life trajectories of "brokers" in AIDS NGOs in Malawi.

11. I do not mean to suggest that these norms of respectable embodiment originated with HIV prevention programs—they drew from standards of middle-class, dominant-caste femininity beyond HIV prevention programs as well. But HIV prevention programs provided a site within which these norms were reinforced.

12. Dickey, "Pleasures and Anxieties," 582.

13. Shobana was threatening to bring the issue up on the agenda at their weekly meeting.

14. The way I heard it, the term *open up* was in English even when the speaker was speaking in Kannada.

15. Benton, *HIV Exceptionalism.*

16. Thanks to Kareem Khubchandani for this observation.

17. Dwaipayan Banerjece points to concealment and nondisclosure as strategies

NOTES TO CHAPTER 5   203

for survival and even circumscribed hope among cancer patients. Banerjee, *Enduring Cancer*, 50. See also Benton, *HIV Exceptionalism*, especially Chapter 3.

18. Lorway and Khan, "Reassembling Epidemiology"; khanna, "Taming of the Shrewd Meyeli Chhele"; and A. Dutta, "Legible Identities and Legitimate Citizens."

19. Supported by the Global Fund, Pehchan is an India-wide program focused on HIV prevention programming for MTH people, channeled through CBOs. The program emphasizes mental health and supportive services beyond HIV testing and promoting condom use. Alliance India, "Pehchan."

20. *Satla-kothi* typically describes a kothi who wears conventionally feminine clothing. *Panthi* typically describes men who play the penetrative role in sex with men (or women). *Jogappas* are a community of gender-fluid men or male women who are dedicated to the goddess Yellamma. Ramberg, *Given to the Goddess*, 35.

21. The word *name* was in English; the rest of the sentence in Kannada.

22. To Alexander, the incident serves an example of how strange the world of HIV prevention is to people like Bill Gates; he describes Gates looking at him in confusion. Alexander, *Stranger Truth*, 156.

23. S. Mohan, *Towards Gender Inclusivity*, 29–31. The authors embed these points within a more complex argument about the politics of naming. They note that funding and NGOs have helped circulate English names with associations that may or may not map onto vernacular practice. At the same time, they note how the lack of indigenous names for certain categories, especially for "female born gender and sexual minorities," has made identification more complicated, and many people opt for English names as simpler than vernacular terms. They also emphasize that "the use of 'Western' terms does not necessarily indicate an acceptance of a Western model of transgender identity" and that "female born gender minorities still find ways to maintain their political agency in accepting these terms."

24. Hubbard, "Sex Zones."

25. Khubchandani's characterization of gay nightlife as generating "small opportunities for radical inclusion, pleasure making, and self-fashioning" is particularly instructive here. Khubchandani, *Ishtyle*, 3.

26. Altman, "Globalization, Political Economy, and HIV/AIDS."

27. A. Gupta, "Blurred Boundaries," 231; Fuller and Harriss, "For an Anthropology," 25; Oldenburg, "Lifestyle as Resistance"; and khanna, "Taming of the Shrewd Meyeli Chhele."

28. Dube, *Indefinite Sentence*, 207. See also M. E. John, "Intersectionality"; Kotiswaran, ed., *Sex Work*; and Kempadoo and Doezema, *Global Sex Workers*.

CHAPTER 6: MAKING IT COUNT

1. The medical sociologist Thurka Sangaramoorthy uses similar accounts of questionnaires being filled out and risk categories documented to show how categories are translated in practice. Categories often do not circulate as intended, and the determination of risk is affected by ideas of racial difference. Sangaramoorthy, "Treating the Numbers."

2. NACO, *Targeted Interventions*, 62.

3. NACO, 274.

4. NACO, 71.

5. Sgaier et al., "Knowing Your HIV/AIDS Epidemic."

6. The package included provision of services (such as STI health services and drop-in centers), outreach and communication (such as peer-led outreach supported by NGOs), community mobilization (including space for community events and training for groups), and creation of an enabling environment (including advocacy and legal education). KHPT, *Pillars of a National HIV Prevention*, 22.

7. Merry, *Seductions of Quantification*, 1.

8. Merry, 21.

9. The travel of quantitative information about India's AIDS response could be thought of as something like Bruno Latour's "immutable mobiles," which "bring celestial bodies billions of tons heavy and hundreds of thousands of miles away to the size of a point on a piece of paper," though this chapter will show that these numbers are mobile but mutable and contested. Latour, *Science in Action*, 227. See also Peck and Theodore, "Mobilizing Policy"; and Sangaramoorthy and Benton, "Enumeration, Identity, and Health."

10. A. Sen, Gates, and Gates, *AIDS Sutra*, 3.

11. Kalpagam, "Colonial State"; and Kalpagam, *Rule by Numbers*.

12. Appadurai, "Number in the Colonial Imagination," 326.

13. Mitra, *Indian Sex Life*.

14. Asad, "Where Are the Margins of the State?"

15. Petryna, "Experimentality"; Nguyen, "Government-by-Exception"; and Rottenburg, "Social and Public Experiments."

16. Fourcade, "State Metrology."

17. Rose, "Governing by Numbers"; and Hansen and Porter, "What Do Numbers Do."

18. Berman and Hirschman, "Sociology of Quantification," 260.

19. Shukla, Teedon, and Cornish, "Empty Rituals?"; Biradavolu et al., "Unintended Consequences"; Lorway, "Making Global Health Knowledge"; and Lorway and Khan, "Reassembling Epidemiology."

20. Peck and Tickell, "Neoliberalizing Space"; and Ganuza and Baiocchi, "Power of Ambiguity."

21. Mudur, "Prevention Proof"; and Associated Press, "Study."

22. Ng et al., "Assessment of Population-Level Effect."

23. Robertson, "Avahan Decade."

24. Gates, "Avahan."

25. Krause, *Good Project*, 2014.

26. Prasada Rao, "Avahan," i7.

27. Avahan's evaluation framework, published in the journal *AIDS* in 2008, noted, "Success for Avahan during its implementation phase is demonstrating that it is possible to build quickly a scaled, quality programme for core and bridge groups across a large geography with complex and heterogeneous local environments." A key expected outcome was to prove this experimentally, as well as to assess its cost-effectiveness. Chandrasekaran et al., "Evaluation Design," S5.

28. Prasada Rao, in "Avahan," describes this change in *success* definition as shifting once the program was underway.

29. For a history of the log-frame as a tool for humanitarian projects, see Chapter 3 of Krause, *The Good Project*.

30. NACO, "NGO/CBO Operational Guidelines," 52–53.

31. The study used the variables of "power within," "power with," and "power over." KHPT, *Evaluation of Community Mobilization*. See also Blanchard et al., "Community Mobilization, Empowerment and HIV."

32. KHPT, *Guidelines for the Formation*, 5.

33. Swidler and Watkins, *Fraught Embrace*; and T. McDonnell, *Best Laid Plans*.

34. Shukla, Teedon, and Cornish, "Empty Rituals?"

35. Chacko, "Chasing Numbers Betraying People."

36. Chacko, 17–18.

37. Baiocchi and Ganuza, "Participatory Budgeting."

38. Shukla, Teedon, and Cornish, "Empty Rituals?"

39. Avahan also funded some impressive efforts to shift the public conversation about AIDS. For example, it sponsored a series of short films related to AIDS and sexuality by prominent directors in Indian languages, and a collection of short stories and essays by well-known Indian writers. A. Sen, Gates, and Gates, *AIDS Sutra*. See also B. Ghosh, "Proximate Truth" for an analysis of the political significance of the 2007 AIDS Jaago films. However, Avahan's own assessments of the impact of its programming in the later years of its tenure in India say much less about these efforts than they do about Avahan's data-driven management practices.

40. Rau, *Avahan-India AIDS Initiative*, 3.

41. Jain, "Gates Gives India More."

42. Alexander, *A Stranger Truth*, 26.

43. Alexander, 264.

44. Alexander, 51.

45. This fact made the Gates Foundation funding different from the USAID funding that dominated the AIDS landscape in much of sub-Saharan Africa and was bound by the Bush-era anti-prostitution pledge.

46. Prasada Rao, "Avahan," i7.

47. Sgaier et al., "How the Avahan HIV Prevention Program Transitioned"; and Prasada Rao, "Avahan."

48. Ng et al., "Assessment of Population-Level Effect."

49. Gates Foundation was also beginning to scale back its funding commitments in global health. Annual reports from the Gates Foundation between 2001 and 2012 indicate that the Gates Foundation was spending 75% of its budget on its global health program in 2001, between 25% and 49% in 2002–2004, and between 59% and 65% in 2005–2011. In 2012, the percentage of funding for global health dropped to 28%. Part of this shift indicated the Foundation's overall interest in reorienting its focus to "global development" rather than global health: in 2012, 49% of the budget went to global development. Gates Foundation, "Annual Reports."

50. Prasada Rao, "Avahan," i7.

51. Prasada Rao, i8.

52. Alexander, *Stranger Truth*, 155.

53. Even in documenting the extent of Avahan's documentation, an emphasis on quantification is clear. Alexander, 265.

54. Sgaier et al., "Knowing Your HIV/AIDS Epidemic," 245.

55. Gates Foundation, "Use It or Lose It," 7.

56. Rau, *Avahan-India AIDS Initiative*, 4.

57. Sgaier et al., "Knowing Your HIV/AIDS Epidemic," 240, 243.

58. Gurnani et al., "Integrated Structural Intervention."

59. Moses et al., "Intensive HIV Prevention."

60. UNAIDS, Global *Report, 2010*, 34.

61. UNAIDS, *Terminology Guidelines*.

62. Robertson, "Avahan Decade."

63. WHO, *Preventing HIV among Sex Workers*, 3.

64. Kerrigan et al., "Global HIV Epidemics."

65. Kerrigan et al., 188. This is the estimate for a program reaching 65% of sex workers.

66. Kerrigan et al., 249.

67. Kerrigan et al., 265.

68. Kerrigan et al., "Community Empowerment."

69. Bridge Project Close-Out Report, 2015.

70. Ashodaya, "Ashodaya Academy."

71. Booth, *Local Women, Global Science.*

72. NACC, *Strategic Plan 2005/6–2009/10*, 13–14.

73. NACC, 22.

74. NACC, 39.

75. NASCOP, *HIV/AIDS*, vii.

76. NASCOP, 5.

77. Pisani et al., "Back to Basics in HIV Prevention"; and Case et al., "Understanding the Modes of Transmission Model."

78. Gelmon et al., "Kenya HIV Prevention Response," vii.

79. Gelmon et al., 15.

80. The report also argued that sex workers were in part at risk because of their "illegal and stigmatized status" and suggested links to a broad range of structural factors: violence, legal structures, war, policy, demographic change, macroeconomic policy, health policy, social policy, illicit drug control policy, poverty, gender inequalities, global capitalism, economic inequalities, racism, sexism, discrimination, and stigmatization. Gelmon et al., 27, 32.

81. Gelmon et al., 39.

82. Mahajan, "Designing Epidemics." Interestingly, Mahajan uses this concept to theorize the use of categories produced in Kenya to study the AIDS epidemic in India in the mid-1980s—a process that was reversed in the mid-2000s.

83. Moral sensitivities also played a role. For example, the Modes of Transmission analysis distinguished between "at-risk populations," like sex workers, who "because of their individual behaviour are at higher risk for transmitting HIV," and "key populations that are vulnerable," such as orphans, "whose situation may lead them to engage in behaviours or subject them to behaviour that may expose them to HIV infection." This distinction allowed subsequent policy to distinguish between those who chose to put themselves at risk and those deserving of programs because their risk was no fault of their own. Gelmon et al., "Kenya HIV Prevention Response," 43.

84. NASCOP, *Kenya AIDS Indicator.*

85. NACC, *Strategic Plan 2009/10–2012/13*, viii.

86. NACC, ix.

87. NACC, xi.

88. NACC, Supporting Documents, 11.

89. NACC, 16.

90. NACC, 24.

91. NACC, 13.

92. NASCOP, *National Guidelines*.

93. NASCOP, 66.

94. NASCOP, 28.

95. NACO, *National AIDS Prevention and Control Policy*, 3.

96. ICRH–Kenya, "About Us."

97. SWOP–Kenya, "Who We Are."

98. BHESP, "About Us."

99. KESWA-Kenya, "About Us."

CHAPTER 7: INDIA IN AFRICA

1. Cornwall, "Buzzwords and Fuzzwords."

2. South-South cooperation, along with *triangular cooperation* (South-South cooperation facilitated by Northern countries, multilateral institutions, or donors), is explicitly mentioned in the 2015 Sustainable Development Goals, and UNDP reports that 15% of its programs and projects utilized South-South or triangular cooperation in 2015.

3. Peck and Theodore, "Recombinant Workfare"; Ganuza and Baiocchi, "Power of Ambiguity"; and Baiocchi and Ganuza, "Participatory Budgeting."

4. Sociologists have theorized the travel of policy and legal norms as *diffusion* processes. Strang and Meyer, "Institutional Conditions for Diffusion"; and Simmons, Dobbin, and Garrett, "Global Diffusion of Public Policies." See also Connell, "Northern Theory of Globalization."

5. Burton, *Africa in the Indian Imagination*, 60.

6. Burton.

7. Go, "Global Fields and Imperial Forms"; Go and Krause, "Fielding Transnationalism"; Buchholz, "What Is a Global Field?"; and Krause, "How Fields Vary."

8. Peck and Theodore, "Mobilizing Policy."

9. Breckenridge, *Biometric State*.

10. Levine, *Prostitution, Race, and Politics*.

11. Burton, *Africa in the Indian Imagination*.

12. See Vahed, "Making of Indianness"; and Radhakrishnan, "Time to Show Our True Colors."

13. Gregory, *India and East Africa*; D. Gupta, "Indian Perceptions of Africa"; Hofmeyr, "Idea of 'Africa'"; and Burton, *Africa in the Indian Imagination*.

14. D. Gupta, "Indian Perceptions of Africa," 162.

15. Burton, *Africa in the Indian Imagination*, 107.

16. Hofmeyr, "Idea of 'Africa,'" 80.

17. D. Gupta, "Indian Perceptions of Africa," 171.

18. Hofmeyr, "Idea of 'Africa,'" 80.

19. McCormick, "China & India"; Naidu, "India's Growing African Strategy"; Narlikar, "India's Rise to Power"; and McCann, "Ties That Bind."

20. See Woods, "Whose Aid?"; and Lee, "Raw Encounters."

21. Naidu, "India's Growing African Strategy," 125.

22. Chorev, "Changing Global Norms."

23. Sindhu, "Modi Doctrine."

24. Carmody, *New Scramble for Africa.*

25. UNAIDS, *Report on the Global AIDS Epidemic,* 2012, A6.

26. UNAIDS, *Global Report,* 2010, 188. In absolute numbers, India's epidemic remained notable—in 2011, Kenya estimated 1.6 million people living with HIV, while India estimated 2.4 million. UNAIDS, *Report on the Global AIDS Epidemic,* 2012, A10; and UNAIDS, *Global Report,* 2010, 187.

27. Baral et al., "Burden of HIV among Female Sex Workers," 541–42.

28. Casarett and Lantos, "Have We Treated AIDS Too Well?"; Benton, *HIV Exceptionalism*; and Morfit, "AIDS Is Money."

29. UNAIDS, *Global Report,* 2010, 236.

30. UNAIDS, 232. For consistency, these figures come from the UNAIDS 2010 *Global Report.* The figures differ slightly from domestic reports. For example, the Kenyan National AIDS Control Council reported a budget of US$629.3 million in 2009–2010, as in NACC, *Kenya National AIDS Strategic Plan 2009/10–2012/13,* 37.

31. These figures come from the OECD CRS. I compiled data for all donors' commitments, including all types of aid. Funding for STD control including HIV/AIDS falls into a different category, population and reproductive health, than the category for health, total, allowing for comparison.

32. According to UNAIDS, similar proportions of AIDS budgets were composed of domestic funds in each country: India contributed 16.5% and Kenya 14.2% (UNAIDS, *Global Report,* 2010, 232, 236). But national reports suggested a different balance of funds.

33. NACC, *Strategic Plan 2009/10–2012/13,* 37.

34. NACO, "Funds and Expenditure."

35. United States Leadership against HIV/AIDS, Tuberculosis, and Malaria Act of 2003, H.R. 1298, 108th Cong. (2003–2004). See also Pai, "Of a Pledge and a People."

36. I calculated these figures from the OECD CRS by compiling funding commitments from the US and from all donors under the category of STD control including HIV/AIDS, in millions of constant 2018 USD.

37. Kenya was a PEPFAR focus country starting in 2004.

38. NACC, *Strategic Plan 2009/10–2012/13*, 37.

39. In addition to directly funding the Avahan program, the Gates Foundation is also the WHO's second largest donor, after the United States, and is also a major donor to the Global Fund to Fight HIV/AIDS, Tuberculosis, and Malaria. Thus, the Gates Foundation's influence is significant to the global AIDS response through multiple pathways. Global Justice Now, *Gated Development*, 10.

40. Pai, "Of a Pledge and a People."

41. In both Kenya and India, laws surrounding sex work are remnants of British law. Neither the Indian Immoral Traffic (Prevention) Act (1986), nor the Indian Penal Code, nor the Kenyan Penal Code, nor the Kenyan Sexual Offences Act (2006) directly criminalizes prostitution—all detail regulation and punishment for activities surrounding prostitution, such as the exploitation of prostitution or living off the earnings of a prostitute. In Kenya, activists point to municipal bylaws as sources of the most frequent arrests, but even the Nairobi General Nuisance By-Laws (2007) criminalize loitering for the purpose of prostitution rather than prostitution itself. In India, too, soliciting for prostitution is criminalized under the Immoral Traffic (Prevention) Act, and sex workers are also booked under public nuisance laws. FIDA Kenya and Open Society Institute, "Documenting Human Rights Violation"; and Mgbako, *To Live Freely*.

42. See White, *The Comforts of Home*, for a discussion of how prostitution was integrated into the fabric of political economy and social relations in colonial Nairobi.

43. A little over half of my interviewees (twelve out of twenty-one in Kenya, and fifty-two out of eighty-two in India) said they felt comfortable identifying publicly as sex workers at least in some contexts.

44. Collins, *Black Sexual Politics*.

45. NASCOP, *HIV/AIDS*, xi.

46. The Kenya Sex Workers' Alliance, in interviews, defined *sex-worker–led organizations* as groups made up of at least 80% current or former sex workers, a percentage higher than that of other local organizations I visited.

47. Seshu, "Collective Courages."

48. A study of HIV prevention programs targeting key populations and drawing on Indian strategies of micro-planning found that it was able to increase the number of contacts peer educators had and the amount of STI screening and HIV testing that took place but that the approach had less of an impact on condom distribution and reporting of violence. Bhattacharjee et al., "Micro-Planning at Scale."

49. Hofmeyr, " Idea of 'Africa,'" 61.

50. Hofmeyr, 61.

CHAPTER 8: AFTER AIDS

1. Deeks, Lewin, and Havlir, "End of AIDS."

2. Sidibé, Piot, and Dybul, "AIDS Is Not Over."

3. "Political Declaration on HIV and AIDS: On the Fast Track to Accelerating the Fight against HIV and to Ending the AIDS Epidemic by 2030," UN General Assembly Res. 70/266 (June 22, 2016). https://www.unaids.org/en/resources/documents/2016/2016-political-declaration-HIV-AIDS.; and UNAIDS, "Miles to Go."

4. Cheng, Juhasz, and Shahani, *AIDS and the Distribution of Crises*, 1.

5. Cheng, Juhasz, and Shahani, 316. See also, in a special issue of *Journal of Medical Humanities*, O'Connell, "Introduction."

6. WHO, "Global Health Estimates 2016."

7. UNAIDS, "Global HIV & AIDS Statistics: 2019 Fact Sheet."

8. Prasada Rao, "Avahan."

9. Sachan, "India's AIDS Department Merger."

10. NACC, *Strategic Plan 2009/10–2012/13*, viii.

11. Jayaraman, "Pool of Infected Women?"

12. World Bank, "World Bank Open Data."

13. Exceptions were Goa, Himachal Pradesh, Kerala, Punjab, and Tamil Nadu.

14. ICMR, PHRI, and IHME, *India*, 33.

15. WHO, "India Taken off WHO's List"; and WHO, "India Three Years Polio-Free."

16. WHO, UNICEF, UNFPA, World Bank, & UNFPA, "Trends in Maternal Mortality." See Say et al., "Global Causes of Maternal Death," e329, for a caveat about how data availability affects this finding.

17. NACO and ICMR, "India HIV Estimations," xxvii.

18. NACO and ICMR, 32.

19. NACO and ICMR, 21, for adults between the ages of fifteen and forty-nine.

20. India was also on track for halving the proportion of the population below the poverty line, eliminating gender disparity in primary and secondary education, and "developing a global partnership for development." It did not meet goals related to maternal mortality, malaria, child mortality, or hunger. UNDP, "Eight Goals for 2015."

21. UN, "Eradicating AIDS."

22. Kerrigan et al., "Global HIV Epidemics," 91.

23. NACO, "National AIDS Control Programme IV."

24. A. Ghosh, "World AIDS Day." She goes on to say, "But now I see the entire programme being destroyed, funds slashed, NACO wound up. I do not know what the future holds."

25. Ghosh.

26. E. McDonnell, "Patchwork Leviathan"; and Paschel, "Disaggregating the Racial State."

27. See Alexander, "Not Just (Any) Body"; Heng, "Great Way to Fly"; Rajan, *Scandal of the State*; Puri, *Sexual States*; and Lakkimsetti, *Legalizing Sex*.

28. Khanna, "Taming of the Shrewd Meyeli Chhele"; Boyce, "Conceiving 'Kothis'"; L. Cohen, "Kothi Wars"; Karnik, "Locating HIV/AIDS and India"; Katyal, *Doubleness of Sexuality*; khanna, *Sexualness*; A. Dutta, "Legible Identities and Legitimate Citizens"; S. Ghosh, "Surveillance in Decolonized Social Space"; Chacko, "Chasing Numbers Betraying People"; ABVA, *Women and AIDS*; ABVA, *Less Than Gay*; and Dube, *Sex, Lies and AIDS*.

29. Kapur, "Postcolonial Erotic Disruptions"; Horton, "Police and the Policed"; khanna, "Social Lives of 377"; and khanna, *Sexualness*.

30. Narrain and Chandra, *Nothing to Fix*.

31. Fassin, *When Bodies Remember*.

32. Calhoun, "World of Emergencies," 376.

33. H. Ghosh, "Under Modi Government."

34. Suresh Kumar Koushal and Another v. Naz Foundation and Others, civil appeal, 10972 of 2013 (India Supreme Court 2013).

35. Puri, *Sexual States*.

36. Chakrabarty, "Section 370"; National Network of Sex Workers, "Clarification Sought."

37. Mandhani, "Anti-Trafficking Bill 2018."

38. Kotiswaran, "Has the Dial Moved?"

39. Navtej Singh Johar and Others v. Union of India, writ petition, 76 of 2016 (India Supreme Court 2018).

40. National Legal Services Authority v. Union of India and Others, writ petition, 400 of 2012, (India Supreme Court 2014).

41. National Network of Sex Workers, "#SexWorkersAdviseHarvardYale"; and Chandra, "Yale to Probe Controversial Study."

42. Lakkimsetti, "Governing Sexualities."

43. Mgbako, *To Live Freely*.

44. Human Rights Watch, "Kenya."

45. A campaign, UN Free and Equal, was launched in 2013.

46. Fassin, *Humanitarian Reason*, xii.

47. Mai, *Mobile Orientations*; and Bernstein, *Brokered Subjects*.

48. Roy, *New South Asian Feminisms*, 19.

49. Cheney, "Gates Foundation COVID-19 Commitment."

50. Gates Foundation, "Annual Reports."

51. Cheney, "Big Concerns." See WHO, "Contributors," for updated data.

52. McGoey, *No Such Thing*; Global Justice Now, *Gated Development*; *The Lancet*, "What Has the Gates Foundation Done?"

53. Roychowdhury, "Delhi Gang Rape."

54. See Prabha Kotiswaran's chapter in Halley et al., *Governance Feminism*; and Kapur, "Gender, Sovereignty and the Rise."

Bibliography

ABVA. *Less Than Gay: A Citizens' Report on the Status of Homosexuality in India.* New Delhi: AIDS Bhedbhav Virodhi Andolan, 1991.

———. *Women and AIDS: Denial and Blame.* New Delhi: AIDS Bhedbhav Virodhi Andolan, 1990.

Agarwala, Rina. *Informal Labor, Formal Politics, and Dignified Discontent in India.* New York: Cambridge University Press, 2013.

AIDS Weekly. "WHO Says Indian AIDS Funds Misused." October 3, 1994.

AIDS Weekly Plus, "India AIDS Situation Seen Out of Control by 2000." *AIDS Weekly Plus*, December 23, 1996, 11–12.

Alexander, Ashok. *A Stranger Truth: Lessons in Love, Leadership and Courage from India's Sex Workers.* New Delhi: Juggernaut Publications, 2018.

Alexander, M. Jacqui. "Not Just (Any) Body Can Be a Citizen: The Politics of Law, Sexuality and Postcoloniality in Trinidad and Tobago and the Bahamas." *Feminist Review* 48, no. 1 (1994): 5–23.

Alliance India. "Pehchan." Alliance India, 2016. http://www.allianceindia.org/our-work/pehchan.

Altman, Dennis. "Globalization, Political Economy, and HIV/AIDS." *Theory and Society* 28, no. 4 (1999): 559–84.

Altman, Lawrence K. "India Suddenly Leads in H.I.V., AIDS Meeting Is Told." *New York Times*, July 8, 1996.

Amar, Paul. *The Security Archipelago: Human-Security States, Sexuality Politics, and the End of Neoliberalism.* Durham, NC: Duke University Press, 2013.

Andrew, Elizabeth W., and Katharine C. Bushnell. *The Queen's Daughters in India*. London: Morgan and Scott, 1898.

Antia, N. H. "AIDS Scare." *Times of India*, November 2, 1995.

Appadurai, Arjun. "Number in the Colonial Imagination." In *Orientalism and the Postcolonial Predicament: Perspectives on South Asia*, edited by Carol A. Breckenridge and Peter van der Veer, 314–39. Philadelphia: University of Pennsylvania Press, 1993.

Aranha, Tina. "Mightier Than the Sword." *DNA India*, January 27, 2006.

Aretxaga, Begoña. "Maddening States." *Annual Review of Anthropology* 32, no. 1 (2003): 393–410.

Armstrong, Elizabeth A., and Mary Bernstein. "Culture, Power, and Institutions: A Multi-Institutional Politics Approach to Social Movements." *Sociological Theory* 26, no. 1 (2008): 74–99.

Arondekar, Anjali. *For the Record: On Sexuality and the Colonial Archive in India*. Durham, NC: Duke University Press, 2009.

Asad, Talal. "Where Are the Margins of the State?" In *Anthropology in the Margins of the State*, edited by Veena Das and Deborah Poole, 279–288. Santa Fe: School of American Research Press, 2004.

Ashodaya Samithi. "Ashodaya Academy." Wings and Initiatives. Accessed 2020. www.ashodayasamithi.org.

Associated Press. "Study: Gates AIDS Project Spared 100K in India." *CBS News*, October 11, 2011.

Asthana, Sheena. "AIDS-Related Policies, Legislation and Programme Implementation in India." *Health Policy and Planning* 11, no. 2 (1996): 184–97.

Atluri, Tara. "The Prerogative of the Brave: Hijras and Sexual Citizenship after Orientalism." *Citizenship Studies* 15, no. 5–6 (2012): 721–36.

Bacchetta, Paola. "When the (Hindu) Nation Exiles Its Queers." *Social Text*, no. 61 (1999): 141–66.

Baiocchi, Gianpaolo, and Ernesto Ganuza. "Participatory Budgeting as If Emancipation Mattered." *Politics & Society* 42, no. 1 (2014): 29–50.

Balogun, Oluwakemi M., and Kimberly Kay Hoang. "Political Economy of Embodiment: Capitalizing on Globally Staged Bodies in Nigerian Beauty Pageants and Vietnamese Sex Work." *Sociological Perspectives* 61, no. 6 (2018): 953–72.

Ban Ki-Moon. "Address to the International AIDS Conference." Presented at the International AIDS Conference, Mexico City, August 3, 2008. https://www.un.org/sg/en/content/sg/speeches/2008-08-03/address-international-aids-conference.

Banerjee, Dwaipayan. *Enduring Cancer: Life, Death, and Diagnosis in Delhi.* Durham, NC: Duke University Press, 2020.

Baral, Stefan, Chris Beyrer, Kathryn Muessig, Tonia Poteat, Andrea L. Wirtz, Michele R. Decker, Susan G. Sherman, and Deanna Kerrigan. "Burden of HIV among Female Sex Workers in Low-Income and Middle-Income Countries: A Systematic Review and Meta-Analysis." *Lancet Infectious Diseases* 12, no. 7 (2012): 538–49.

Bardhan, Pranab, Sandip Mitra, Dilip Mookherjee, and Anusha Nath. "Changing Voting Patterns in Rural West Bengal." *Economic & Political Weekly* 49, no. 11 (2014): 55.

Bartlett, J. G. "AIDS in India." *Medicine* 74, no. 2 (March 1995): 107–8.

Beck, Ulrich. *World at Risk.* Malden, MA: Polity, 2009.

Benjamin, Solomon. "Governance, Economic Settings and Poverty in Bangalore." *Environment and Urbanization* 12, no. 1 (2000): 35–56.

Benton, Adia. *HIV Exceptionalism: Development through Disease in Sierra Leone.* Minneapolis: University of Minnesota Press, 2015.

Berlant, Lauren. "Slow Death (Sovereignty, Obesity, Lateral Agency)." *Critical Inquiry* 33, no. 4 (2007): 754–80.

Berman, Elizabeth Popp, and Daniel Hirschman. "The Sociology of Quantification: Where Are We Now?" *Contemporary Sociology* 47, no. 3 (2018): 257–66.

Bernstein, Elizabeth. *Brokered Subjects: Sex, Trafficking, and the Politics of Freedom.* Chicago: University of Chicago Press, 2018.

Berry, Marie E. *War, Women, and Power: From Violence to Mobilization in Rwanda and Bosnia-Herzegovina.* Cambridge University Press, 2018.

Bhambra, Gurminder K. "Comparative Historical Sociology and the State: Problems of Method." *Cultural Sociology* 10, no. 3 (2016): 335–51.

Bhargava, Simran, and David Devadas. "People Say There Is a Lot of Sex on Campus: A.S. Paintal." *India Today*, July 31, 1988.

Bhaskaran, Suparna. "The Politics of Penetration: Section 377 of the Indian Penal Code." In *Queering India: Same-Sex Love and Eroticism in Indian Culture and Society*, edited by Ruth Vanita, 15–29. New York: Routledge, 2002.

Bhattacharjee, Parinita, Helgar Musyoki, Ravi Prakash, Serah Malaba, Gina Dallabetta, Tisha Wheeler, Stephen Moses, Shajy Isac, and Richard Steen. "Micro-Planning at Scale with Key Populations in Kenya: Optimising Peer Educator Ratios for Programme Outreach and HIV/STI Service Utilisation." *PLoS ONE* 13, no. 11 (2018).

BHESP. "About Us." Bar Hostesses Empowerment and Support Programme. Accessed 2020. https://www.bhesp.org/index.php/2016-02-29-10-29-39.

Biehl, João. "The Activist State: Global Pharmaceuticals, AIDS and Citizenship in Brazil." *Social Text* 22, no. 3 (2004): 105–32.

———. *Will to Live: AIDS Therapies and the Politics of Survival*. Princeton, NJ: Princeton University Press, 2007.

Biradavolu, Monica, Kim Blankenship, Annie George, and Nimesh Dhungana. "Unintended Consequences of Community-Based Monitoring Systems: Lessons for an HIV Prevention Intervention for Sex Workers in South India." *World Development* 67 (2015): 1–10.

Blanchard, Andrea K., Haranahalli Lakkappa Mohan, Maryam Shahmanesh, Ravi Prakash, Shajy Isac, Banadakoppa Manjappa Ramesh, Parinita Bhattacharjee, Vandana Gurnani, Stephen Moses, and James F. Blanchard. "Community Mobilization, Empowerment and HIV Prevention among Female Sex Workers in South India." *BMC Public Health* 13, no. 1 (2013): 234.

Blankenship, Kim, Monica Biradavolu, Asima Jena, and Annie George. "Challenging the Stigmatization of Female Sex Workers through a Community-Led Structural Intervention: Learning from a Case Study of a Female Sex Worker Intervention in Andhra Pradesh, India." *AIDS Care* 22, no. S2 (2010): 1629–36.

Bollinger, R. C., S. P. Tripathy, and T. C. Quinn. "The Human Immunodeficiency Virus Epidemic in India. Current Magnitude and Future Projections." *Medicine* 74, no. 2 (1995): 97–106.

Booth, Karen M. *Local Women, Global Science: Fighting AIDS in Kenya*. Bloomington: Indiana University Press, 2004.

Bourdieu, Pierre, and Loïc Wacquant. *An Invitation to Reflexive Sociology*. Chicago: University of Chicago Press, 1992.

Boyce, Paul. "Conceiving 'Kothis': Men Who Have Sex with Men in India and the Cultural Subject of HIV Prevention." *Medical Anthropology* 26, no. 2 (2007): 175–203.

Boyce, Paul, and akshay khanna. "Rights and Representations: Querying the Male-to-Male Sexual Subject in India." *Culture, Health & Sexuality* 13, no. 1 (2011): 89–100.

Breckenridge, Keith. *Biometric State: The Global Politics of Identification and Surveillance in South Africa, 1850 to the Present*. Cambridge, UK: Cambridge University Press, 2014.

Brookmeyer, R., T. Quinn, M. Shepherd, S. Mehendale, J. Rodrigues, and R. Bollinger. "The AIDS Epidemic in India: A New Method for Estimating Current Human Immunodeficiency Virus (HIV) Incidence Rates." *American Journal of Epidemiology* 142, no. 7 (1995): 709–13.

Brown, Wendy. "Finding the Man in the State." *Feminist Studies* 18, no. 1 (1992): 7–34.

Buchholz, Larissa. "What Is a Global Field? Theorizing Fields beyond the Nation-State." *Sociological Review* 64, no. 2 (2016): 31–60.

Burawoy, Michael. *Global Ethnography*. Berkeley: University of California Press, 2000.

———."Manufacturing the Global." *Ethnography* 2, no. 2 (2001): 147–59.

Burns, John F. "Denial and Taboo Blinding India to the Horror of Its AIDS Scourge." *New York Times*, September 22, 1996.

Burton, Antoinette. *Africa in the Indian Imagination: Race and the Politics of Postcolonial Citation*. Durham, NC: Duke University Press, 2016.

Burton, Antoinette M. *Burdens of History: British Feminists, Indian Women, and Imperial Culture, 1865–1915*. Chapel Hill: University of North Carolina Press, 1994.

CAG. *Union Government (Civil) Performance Appraisals (3 of 2004) on National AIDS Control Programme (Ministry of Health and Family Welfare)*. New Delhi: Comptroller and Auditor General of India, 2003.

Calhoun, Craig. "A World of Emergencies: Fear, Intervention, and the Limits of Cosmopolitan Order." *Canadian Review of Sociology / Revue Canadienne de Sociologie* 41, no. 4 (2004): 373–95.

Campbell, Catherine. *Letting Them Die: Why HIV/AIDS Intervention Programmes Fail*. Bloomington: Indiana University Press, 2003.

Carmody, Pádraig. *The New Scramble for Africa*. Malden, MA: Polity, 2011.

Carrillo, Héctor. *The Night Is Young: Sexuality in Mexico in the Time of AIDS*. Chicago: University of Chicago Press, 2002.

Casarett, David, and John Lantos. "Have We Treated AIDS Too Well? Rationing and the Future of AIDS Exceptionalism." *Annals of Internal Medicine* 128, no. 9 (1998): 756–59.

Case, Kelsey K., Peter D. Ghys, Eleanor Gouws, Jeffrey W. Eaton, Annick Borquez, John Stover, Paloma Cuchi, Laith J. Abu-Raddad, Geoffrey P. Garnett, and Timothy B. Hallett. "Understanding the Modes of Transmission Model of New HIV Infection and Its Use in Prevention Planning." *Bulletin of the World Health Organization* 90, no. 11 (2012): 831–38.

Center for Advocacy on Stigma and Marginalisation. *Rights-Based Sex Worker Empowerment Guidelines: An Alternative HIV/AIDS Intervention Approach to the 100% Condom Use Program*. Sangli: SANGRAM, 2008.

Chacko, Shubha. *Chasing Numbers Betraying People: Relooking at HIV Related Services in Karnataka*. Bangalore: Aneka, 2011.

Chakrabarty, Rakhi. "Section 370 Not for Voluntary Sex Work: Verma Panel." *Times of India*, February 12, 2013.

Chandra, Jagriti. "Yale to Probe Controversial Study on Sex Workers." *The Hindu*, July 9, 2020.

Chandrasekaran, Padma, Gina Dallabetta, Virginia Loo, Stephen Mills, Tobi Saidel, Rajatashuvra Adhikary, Michel Alary, Catherine M. Lowndes, Marie-Claude Boily, and James Moore. "Evaluation Design for Large-Scale HIV Prevention Programmes: The Case of Avahan, the India AIDS Initiative." *AIDS* 22 (2008): S1–S15.

Chatterjee, Patralekha. "AIDS in India: Police Powers and Public Health." *Lancet* 367, no. 9513 (2006): 805–6.

Cheney, Catherine. "Gates Foundation COVID-19 Commitment Reaches $1.75B with Latest Pledge." *DevEx*, December 10, 2020.

———. "'Big Concerns' over Gates Foundation's Potential to Become Largest WHO Donor." *DevEx*, June 5, 2020.

Cheng, Jih-Fei, Alexandra Juhasz, and Nishant Shahani. *AIDS and the Distribution of Crises*. Durham, NC: Duke University Press, 2020.

Chin, James, and Alan Gillies. *The AIDS Pandemic: The Collision of Epidemiology with Political Correctness*. Seattle: Radcliffe Publishing, 2006.

Chin, James, P. A. Sato, and Jonathan M. Mann. "Projections of HIV Infections and AIDS Cases to the Year 2000." *Bulletin of the World Health Organization* 68, no. 1 (1990): 1.

Chitre, Ajit. "AIDS Mania." *Times of India*, January 11, 1990.

Chorev, Nitsan. "Changing Global Norms through Reactive Diffusion: The Case of Intellectual Property Protection of AIDS Drugs." *American Sociological Review* 77, no. 5 (2012): 831–53.

———. *Give and Take: Developmental Foreign Aid and the Pharmaceutical Industry in East Africa*. Princeton, NJ: Princeton University Press, 2019.

Chowdhury, A. N. "AIDS Prevention: What Are We Talking About?" *Journal of the Indian Medical Association* 89, no. 11 (1991): 304–5.

Cohen, Cathy. *The Boundaries of Blackness: AIDS and the Breakdown of Black Politics*. Chicago: University of Chicago Press, 1999.

Cohen, Lawrence. "The Kothi Wars: AIDS Cosmopolitanism and the Morality of Classification." In *Sex in Development: Science, Sexuality, and Morality in Global Perspective*, edited by Stacy Leigh Pigg and Vincanne Adams, 269–303. Durham, NC: Duke University Press, 2005.

———. "Song for Pushkin." *Daedalus* 136, no. 2 (2007): 103–15.

Collins, Patricia Hill. *Black Sexual Politics: African Americans, Gender, and the New Racism*. New York: Routledge, 2004.

Comaroff, Jean. "Beyond Bare Life: AIDS, (Bio)Politics, and the Neoliberal Order." *Public Culture* 19, no. 1 (2007): 197–219.

Connell, Raewyn. "The Northern Theory of Globalization." *Sociological Theory* 25, no. 4 (2007): 368–85.

——. "The State, Gender, and Sexual Politics: Theory and Appraisal." *Theory and Society* 19, no. 5 (1990): 507–44.

Cooper, Davina. "An Engaged State: Sexuality, Governance, and the Potential for Change." *Journal of Law and Society* 20, no. 3 (1993): 257–75.

Cooper, Frederic. "Writing the History of Development." *Journal of Modern European History* 8, no. 1 (2010): 5–23.

Cornwall, Andrea. "Buzzwords and Fuzzwords: Deconstructing Development Discourse." *Development in Practice* 17, no. 4–5 (2007): 471–84.

Dalal, Gaurang B. "AIDS Bomb." *Times of India*, November 14, 1995.

Dancy-Scott, Nicole, Gale A. Dutcher, Alla Keselman, Colette Hochstein, Christina Copty, Diane Ben-Senia, Sampada Rajan, et al. "Trends in HIV Terminology: Text Mining and Data Visualization Assessment of International AIDS Conference Abstracts over 25 Years." *JMIR Public Health and Surveillance* 4, no. 2 (2018).

Dandona, Lalit, Rakhi Dandona, Juan Pablo Gutierrez, G. Anil Kumar, Sam McPherson, Stefano M. Bertozzi, and ASCI FPP Study Team. "Sex Behaviour of Men Who Have Sex with Men and Risk of HIV in Andhra Pradesh, India." *AIDS* 19, no. 6 (2005): 611–19.

Dandona, Lalit, Vemu Lakshmi, G. Anil Kumar, and Rakhi Dandona. "Is the HIV Burden in India Being Overestimated?" *BMC Public Health* 6 (2006): 308.

Dasgupta, Simanti. "Of Raids and Returns: Sex Work Movement, Police Oppression, and the Politics of the Ordinary in Sonagachi, India." *Anti-Trafficking Review*, no. 12 (2019): 127–39.

D'Costa, Lourdes J., Francis A. Plummer, Ian Bowmer, Lieve Fransen, Peter Piot, Allan R. Ronald, and Herbert Nsanze. "Prostitutes Are a Major Reservoir of Sexually Transmitted Diseases in Nairobi, Kenya." *Sexually Transmitted Diseases* 12, no. 2 (1985): 64–67.

Decoteau, Claire Laurier. *Ancestors and Antiretrovirals: The Biopolitics of HIV/AIDS in Post-Apartheid South Africa*. Chicago: University of Chicago Press, 2013.

——. "Exclusionary Inclusion and the Normalization of Biomedical Culture." *American Journal of Cultural Sociology* 1, no. 3 (2013): 403–30.

Deeks, Steven G., Sharon R. Lewin, and Diane V. Havlir. "The End of AIDS: HIV Infection as a Chronic Disease." *Lancet* 382, no. 9903 (2013): 1525–33.

De Souza, Rebecca. "The Construction of HIV/AIDS in Indian Newspapers: A Frame Analysis." *Health Communication* 21, no. 3 (2007): 257–66.

Dhingra, Neeraj, Prabhat Jha, Vinod P. Sharma, Alan A. Cohen, Raju M. Jotkar, Peter S. Rodriguez, Diego G. Bassani, Wilson Suraweera, Ramanan Laxminarayan, and Richard Peto. "Adult and Child Malaria Mortality in India." *Lancet* 376, no. 9754 (2010): 1768–74.

Dickey, Sara. "The Pleasures and Anxieties of Being in the Middle: Emerging Middle-Class Identities in Urban South India." *Modern Asian Studies* 46, no. 3 (2012): 559–99.

DMSC. "Durbar Mahila Samanwaya Committee." Accessed 2017. www.durbar.org.

———. "Sex Workers' Manifesto." Kolkata: Durbar Mahila Samanwaya Committee, 1997.

Doezema, Jo. "Ouch!: Western Feminists' 'Wounded Attachment' to the 'Third World Prostitute.'" *Feminist Review* 67 (2001): 16–38.

Dube, Siddharth. *An Indefinite Sentence: A Personal History of Outlawed Love and Sex*. New York: Simon and Schuster, 2019.

———. *Sex, Lies and AIDS*. New Delhi: HarperCollins Publishers India, 1997.

Duggan, Lisa. "Queering the State." *Social Text*, no. 39 (1994): 1–14.

Dutta, Aniruddha. "Legible Identities and Legitimate Citizens: The Globalization of Transgender and Subjects of HIV-AIDS Prevention in Eastern India." *International Feminist Journal of Politics* 15, no. 4 (2013): 494–514.

Dutta, G. P. "Problems of AIDS in Developing Countries." *Journal of the Indian Medical Association* 90, no. 10 (1992): 254–56.

Eberstadt, Nicholas. "The Future of AIDS." *Foreign Affairs*, December 2002, 22–45.

Enloe, Cynthia. *Bananas, Beaches and Bases: Making Feminist Sense of International Politics*. Berkeley: University of California Press, 2014.

Epstein, Steven. *Impure Science: AIDS, Activism, and the Politics of Knowledge*. Berkeley: University of California Press, 1996.

Escobar, Arturo. "Place, Nature and Culture in Discourses of Globalization." In *Localizing Knowledge in a Globalizing World: Recasting the Area Studies Debate*, edited by Ali Mirsepassi, Amrita Basu, and Frederick Weaver, 37–59. Syracuse: Syracuse University Press, 2003.

Euser, Sjoerd, Dennis Souverein, Pushpalatha Rama Narayana Gowda, Chandra Shekhar Gowda, Diana Grootendorst, Rajendra Ramaiah, Snehal Barot, et al. "Pragati: An Empowerment Programme for Female Sex Workers in Bangalore, India." *Global Health Action* 5, no. 1 (2012): 1–11.

Evans, Peter. *Embedded Autonomy: States and Industrial Transformation*. Princeton, NJ: Princeton University Press, 1995.

Evans, Peter, and Patrick Heller. "The State and Development." In *Asian Transformations: An Inquiry into the Development of Nations*, edited by Deepak Nayyar, 109–35. Oxford, UK: Oxford University Press, 2019.

Farmer, Paul. *AIDS and Accusation: Haiti and the Geography of Blame*. Berkeley: University of California Press, 1990.

———. *Infections and Inequalities: The Modern Plagues*. Berkeley: University of California Press, 2001.

Fassin, Didier. *Humanitarian Reason: A Moral History of the Present*. Berkeley: University of California Press, 2011.

———. *When Bodies Remember: Experiences and Politics of AIDS in South Africa*. Berkeley: University of California Press, 2007.

Ferguson, James, and Akhil Gupta. "Spatializing States: Toward an Ethnography of Neoliberal Governmentality." *American Ethnologist* 29, no. 4 (2002): 981–1002.

FIDA Kenya and Open Society Institute. "Documenting Human Rights Violation of Sex Workers in Kenya." Nairobi: FIDA Kenya and Open Society Institute, 2008.

Fourcade, Marion. "State Metrology: The Rating of Sovereigns and the Judgment of Nations." In *The Many Hands of the State: Theorizing Political Authority and Social Control*, edited by Kimberly J. Morgan and Ann Shola Orloff, 103–27. New York: Cambridge University Press, 2017.

Friedman, Thomas. "Bangalore: Hot and Hotter." Opinion, *New York Times*, June 8, 2005.

Fuller, Chris, and John Harriss. "For an Anthropology of the Modern Indian State." In *The Everyday State and Society in Modern India*, edited by Chris Fuller and Veronique Benei, 1–30. London: Hurst & Co, 2001.

Ganuza, Ernesto, and Gianpaolo Baiocchi. "The Power of Ambiguity: How Participatory Budgeting Travels the Globe." *Journal of Public Deliberation* 8, no. 2 (2012): 1–12.

Gates, Bill. "Avahan: Winning against HIV/AIDS in India." *Gates Notes* (blog), 2012. www.gatesnotes.com/Health/Avahan-Winning-Against-HIV-AIDS-in-India.

Gates Foundation. "Use It or Lose It: How Avahan Used Data to Shape Its HIV Prevention Efforts in India." New Delhi: Bill & Melinda Gates Foundation, 2008.

———. "Annual Reports." https://www.gatesfoundation.org/Who-We-Are/Resources-and-Media/Annual-Reports.

Gelmon, Lawrence, Patrick Kenya, Francis Oguya, Boaz Cheluget, and Girmay Haile. "Kenya HIV Prevention Response and Modes of Transmission Analysis." Nairobi: National AIDS Control Council, 2009.

Ghosh, Abantika. "World AIDS Day: India Slashes Aid to Programme after Major Success Fighting It." *Indian Express*, December 1, 2015.

Ghosh, Bishnupriya. "The Costs of Living: Reflections on Global Health Crises."

In *AIDS and the Distribution of Crises*, edited by Jih-Fei Cheng, Alexandra Juhasz, and Nishant Shahani. Durham, NC: Duke University Press, 2020.

———. "The Proximate Truth: Reenactment in the Pandemic-Era HIV/AIDS Documentaries." *BioScope: South Asian Screen Studies* 3, no. 1 (2012): 69–86.

Ghosh, Himadri. "Under Modi Government, Foreign Funding of NGOs Has Come Down." NewsLaundry, May 20, 2016.

Ghosh, Swati. "Elusive Choice and Agency: A Feminist Re-Reading of the Sex Workers' Manifesto." In *Prostitution and Beyond: AIn Analysis of Sex Workers in India*, by Rohini Sahni and V. Kalyan Shankar. New Delhi: Sage, 2008.

———. *The Gendered Proletariat: Sex Work, Workers' Movement, and Agency*. New Delhi: Oxford University Press India, 2018.

———. "Surveillance in Decolonized Social Space: The Case of Sex Workers in Bengal." *Social Text* 23, no. 2 (2005): 55.

Ghosh, T. K. "AIDS: A Serious Challenge to Public Health." *Journal of the Indian Medical Association* 84, no. 1 (1986): 29.

Gilada, I. S. Response to "Doctor in India arrested over irregularities trial of vaccine" by Mudur Ganapati. *BMJ* 318 (1999): 1308.

Global Justice Now. *Gated Development: Is the Gates Foundation Always a Force for Good?* London: Global Justice Now, 2016.

Go, Julian. "Global Fields and Imperial Forms: Field Theory and the British and American Empires." *Sociological Theory* 26, no. 3 (2008): 201–29.

———. *Postcolonial Thought and Social Theory*. New York: Oxford University Press, 2016.

Go, Julian, and Monika Krause. "Fielding Transnationalism: An Introduction." *Sociological Review Monographs* 64, no. 2 (2016): 6–30.

Gooptu, Nandini, and Nandinee Bandyopadhyay. "'Rights to Stop the Wrong': Cultural Change and Collective Mobilization—The Case of Kolkata Sex Workers." *Oxford Development Studies* 35, no. 3 (2007): 251–72.

Gopal, Meena. "Ruptures and Reproduction in Caste/Gender/Labour." *Economic and Political Weekly* 48, no. 18 (2013): 91–97.

Gould, Deborah. *Moving Politics: Emotion and ACT UP's Fight against AIDS*. Chicago: University of Chicago Press, 2009.

Gregory, Robert G. *India and East Africa: A History of Race Relations within the British Empire, 1890–1939*. Oxford, UK: Clarendon Press, 1971.

Grewal, Inderpal. *Transnational America: Feminisms, Diasporas, Neoliberalisms*. Durham, NC: Duke University Press, 2005.

Grewal, Inderpal, and Caren Kaplan. *Scattered Hegemonies: Postmodernity and Transnational Feminist Practices*. Minneapolis: University of Minnesota Press, 1994.

Gupta, Akhil. "Blurred Boundaries: The Discourse of Corruption, the Culture of Politics, and the Imagined State." *American Ethnologist* 22, no. 2 (1995): 375–402.

———. *Red Tape: Bureaucracy, Structural Violence, and Poverty in India*. Durham, NC: Duke University Press, 2012.

Gupta, Dhruba. "Indian Perceptions of Africa." *South Asia Research* 11, no. 2 (1991): 158–74.

Gupta, Ruchira. "In Kolkata, Reminders of Why We Help the 'Last Girl.'" *New York Times*, March 7, 2014.

Gurnani, Vandana, Tara S. Beattie, Parinita Bhattacharjee, H. L. Mohan, Srinath Maddur, Reynold Washington, Shajy Isac, B. M. Ramesh, Stephen Moses, and James F. Blanchard. "An Integrated Structural Intervention to Reduce Vulnerability to HIV and Sexually Transmitted Infections among Female Sex Workers in Karnataka State, South India." *BMC Public Health* 11, no. 1 (2011): 755.

Hall, Stuart. *Cultural Studies 1983: A Theoretical History*. Durham, NC: Duke University Press, 2016.

———. "Cultural Studies and Its Theoretical Legacies." In *Cultural Studies*, edited by Lawrence Grossberg, Cary Nelson, and Paula Treichler, 277–94. New York: Routledge, 1992.

Halley, Janet, Prabha Kotiswaran, Rachel Rebouché, and Hila Shamir. *Governance Feminism: An Introduction*. Minneapolis: University of Minnesota Press, 2018.

Hansen, Hans Krause, and Tony Porter. "What Do Numbers Do in Transnational Governance?" *International Political Sociology* 6, no. 4 (2012): 409–26.

Hansen, Thomas Blom, Finn Stepputat, Julia Adams, and George Steinmetz. *States of Imagination: Ethnographic Explorations of the Postcolonial State*. Durham, NC: Duke University Press, 2001.

Harris, Joseph. *Achieving Access: Professional Movements and the Politics of Health Universalism*. Ithaca, NY: Cornell University Press, 2017.

Hart, Gillian. *Disabling Globalization: Places of Power in Post-Apartheid South Africa*. Berkeley: University of California Press, 2002.

Hazarika, Sanjoy. "In an Unaware India, AIDS Threat Is Growing." *New York Times*, August 9, 1990.

———. "To Fight AIDS, Indian Urges Ban on Sex with Foreigners." *New York Times*, June 15, 1988.

Heng, Geraldine. "'A Great Way to Fly': Nationalism, the State, and the Varieties of Third-World Feminism." In *Feminist Genealogies, Colonial Legacies, Democratic Futures*, edited by M. Jacqui Alexander and Chandra Talpade Mohanty, 30–45. New York: Routledge, 1996.

The Hindu. "Pension Parishad Campaign in Bangalore Today." August 9, 2012.

Hodge, Joseph. "British Colonial Expertise, Post-Colonial Careering and the Early History of International Development." *Journal of Modern European History* 8, no. 1 (2010): 24–46.

Hodges, Sarah. "'Looting' the Lock Hospital in Colonial Madras during the Famine Years of the 1870s." *Social History of Medicine* 18, no. 3 (2005): 379–98.

Hofmeyr, Isabel. "The Idea of 'Africa' in Indian Nationalism: Reporting the Diaspora in *The Modern Review* 1907–1929." *South African Historical Journal* 57, no. 1 (2007): 60–81.

Holt, Richard. "Global Cities: Which Cities Will Be Leading the Global Economy in 2035?" Oxford, UK: Oxford Economics, 2018.

Horton, Brian. "The Police and the Policed: Queer Crossings in a Bombay Bathroom." In *Queer Nightlife*, edited by Ramon H. Rivera-Servera, Kemi Adeyemi, and Kareem Khubchandani. Ann Arbor: University of Michigan Press, forthcoming.

Hubbard, Phil. "Sex Zones: Intimacy, Citizenship and Public Space." *Sexualities* 4, no. 1 (2001): 51–71.

Hull, Matthew S. *Government of Paper: The Materiality of Bureaucracy in Urban Pakistan.* Berkeley: University of California Press, 2012.

Human Rights Watch. *Epidemic of Abuse: Police Harassment of HIV/AIDS Outreach Workers in India.* New Delhi: Human Rights Watch, 2002.

———."India: Confirm Policy Ending Mandatory HIV Tests." July 21, 2012. https://www.hrw.org/news/2012/07/21/india-confirm-policy-ending-mandatory-hiv-tests.

———."Kenya: Court Upholds Archaic Anti-Homosexuality Laws." LGBT Rights. May 24, 2019. https://www.hrw.org/news/2019/05/24/kenya-court-upholds-archaic-anti-homosexuality-laws.

Humsafar Trust. "About Us." Accessed 2019. https://humsafar.org/.

Hunter, Mark. "Beyond the Male-Migrant: South Africa's Long History of Health Geography and the Contemporary AIDS Pandemic." *Health & Place* 16, no. 1 (2010): 25–33.

———.*Love in the Time of AIDS: Inequality, Gender, and Rights in South Africa.* Bloomington: Indiana University Press, 2010.

———."The Materiality of Everyday Sex: Thinking beyond 'Prostitution.'" *African Studies* 61, no. 1 (2002): 99–120.

ICMR, PHRI, and IHME. *India: Health of the Nation's States: The India State-Level Disease Burden Initiative.* New Delhi: Indian Council of Medical Research, Public Health Foundation of India, and Institute for Health Metrics and Evaluation, 2017.

ICRH–Kenya. "About Us." International Centre for Reproductive Health–Kenya. Accessed September 8, 2020. https://www.icrhk.org/.

Imam, Zaka. "India's AIDS Control Programme Is Unsatisfactory." *British Medical Journal* 308, no. 6933 (1994): 873–78.

Inderjit, Sabina. "Even Hospitals Reject AIDS Patients." *Times of India*, July 19, 1990.

India Today, "India's AIDS Control Mission a Successful Model." *India Today*. February 8, 2012.

Inglis, Patrick. *Narrow Fairways: Getting By & Falling Behind in the New India.* New York: Oxford University Press, 2019.

Jain, Kalpana. "Gates Gives India More Than Africa for AIDS." *Times of India*, November 12, 2002.

Jana, Smarajit, Ishika Basu, Mary Jane Rotheram-Borus, and Peter A. Newman. "The Sonagachi Project: A Sustainable Community Intervention Program." *AIDS Education and Prevention* 16, no. 5 (2004): 405–14.

Jayadeva, Sazana. "'Below English Line': An Ethnographic Exploration of Class and the English Language in Post-Liberalization India." *Modern Asian Studies* 52, no. 2 (2018): 576–608.

Jayaraman, K. S. "AIDS in Position to Ravage India." *Nature Medicine* 2, no. 9 (1996): 951.

———. "AIDS Institute for India?" *Nature* 326, no. 6111 (1987): 322.

———. "Disaster Looms for Bombay." *Nature* 346 (1990): 499.

———. "Drastic Measures Proposed in India." *Nature* 333, no. 6175 (1988): 697.

———. "India against AIDS." *Nature* 318, no. 201 (1985).

———. "India Screens Foreign Students for AIDS." *Nature* 324, no. 6095 (1986): 194.

———. "Pool of Infected Women? AIDS in India." *Nature* 321, no. 6066 (1986): 103.

———. "Students in India Object to AIDS Test." *Nature* 326, no. 6108 (1987): 4.

Jayaraman, K. S., and C. Macilwain. "India Moves Ahead Cautiously on US AIDS Project." *Nature* 363, no. 6427 (1993): 294.

Jenkins, Carol. *Female Sex Worker HIV Prevention Projects: Lessons Learnt from Papua New Guinea, India and Bangladesh.* Geneva: UNAIDS, 2000.

Jha, Prabhat, Rajesh Kumar, Ajay Khera, Madhulekha Bhattacharya, Paul Arora, Vendhan Gajalakshmi, Prakash Bhatia, et al. "HIV Mortality and Infection in India: Estimates from Nationally Representative Mortality Survey of 1.1 Million Homes." *BMJ* 340, no. c621 (2010).

John, Mary E. "Intersectionality: Rejection or Critical Dialogue?" *Economic and Political Weekly* 50, no. 33 (2015): 72–76.

John, T. Jacob, P. George Babu, Harriet Jayakumari, and E. A. Simoes. "Prevalence of HIV Infection in Risk Groups in Tamil Nadu, India." *Lancet* 1, no. 8525 (1987): 160.

Johnston, Timothy, and Martha Ainsworth. "Project Performance Assessment Report, India, National AIDS Control Project (Credit No. 2350)." Washington, DC: Sector and Thematic Evaluation Group, Operations Evaluation Department, World Bank, 2003.

Kadri, A. M., and Pradeep Kumar. "Institutionalization of the NACP and Way Ahead." *Indian Journal of Community Medicine* 37, no. 2 (2012): 83–88.

Kalpagam, U. "The Colonial State and Statistical Knowledge." *History of the Human Sciences* 13, no. 2 (2000): 37–55.

———.*Rule by Numbers: Governmentality in Colonial India*. Lanham, Maryland: Lexington Books, 2014.

Kang, Bhavdeep. "India May Face an Africa-like AIDS Situation." *The Pioneer*, October 13, 1992.

Kannabiran, Kalpana. "Judiciary, Social Reform and Debate on 'Religious Prostitution' in Colonial India." *Economic and Political Weekly* 30, no. 43 (1995): WS59–69.

Kapur, Ratna. "The Citizen and the Migrant: Postcolonial Anxieties, Law, and the Politics of Exclusion/Inclusion." *Theoretical Inquiries in Law* 8, no. 2 (2007): 537–70.

———. "Gender, Sovereignty and the Rise of Sexual Security Regime in International Law and Postcolonial India." *Melbourne Journal of International Law* 14 (2013): 317.

———. "Postcolonial Erotic Disruptions: Legal Narratives of Culture, Sex, and Nation in India." *Columbia Journal of Gender and Law* 10, no. 2 (2001).

Karnik, Niranjan. "Locating HIV/AIDS and India: Cautionary Notes on the Globalization of Categories." *Science, Technology & Human Values* 26, no. 3 (2001): 322–48.

Katyal, Akhil. *The Doubleness of Sexuality: Idioms of Same-Sex Desire in Modern India*. New Delhi: New Text, 2016.

Keck, Margaret E., and Kathryn Sikkink. *Activists beyond Borders: Advocacy Networks in International Politics*. Ithaca: Cornell University Press, 1998.

Kempadoo, Kamala. *Sexing the Caribbean: Gender, Race and Sexual Labor*. New York: Routledge, 2004.

Kempadoo, Kamala, and Jo Doezema. *Global Sex Workers: Rights, Resistance, and Redefinition*. New York: Routledge, 1998.

Kerrigan, Deanna, Virginia Fonner, Susanne Stromdahl, and Caitlin Kennedy.

"Community Empowerment among Female Sex Workers Is an Effective HIV Prevention Intervention: A Systematic Review of the Peer-Reviewed Evidence from Low- and Middle-Income Countries." *AIDS and Behavior* 17, no. 6 (2013): 1926–40.

Kerrigan, Deanna, Andrea Wirtz, Stefan Baral, Michele Decker, Laura Murray, Tonia Poteat, Carel Pretorius, et al. "The Global HIV Epidemics among Sex Workers." Washington, DC: World Bank, 2013.

KESWA-Kenya. "About Us." KESWA-Kenya, 2019. https://keswa-kenya.org/about-us/.

Khan, Shivananda. "Culture, Sexualities, and Identities: Men Who Have Sex with Men in India." *Journal of Homosexuality* 40, no. 3–4 (2001): 99–115.

khanna, akshay. *Sexualness*. New Delhi: New Text, 2016.

———. "The Social Lives of 377: Constitution of the Law by the Queer Movement." In *Law Like Love: Queer Perspectives on the Law*, edited by Gautam Bhan and Arvind Narrain, 174–202. New Delhi: Yoda Press, 2011.

———. "Taming of the Shrewd Meyeli Chhele: A Political Economy of Development's Sexual Subject." *Development* 52, no. 1 (2009): 43–51.

KHPT. *Evaluation of Community Mobilization*. Bangalore: Karnataka Health Promotion Trust, 2012.

———. *Guidelines for the Formation of Collectives of Women in Sex Work and Their Administration*. Bangalore: Karnataka Health Promotion Trust, 2009.

———. *The Pillars of a National HIV Prevention Response: A Guide for National Program Managers*. Bangalore: Karnataka Health Promotion Trust, 2013.

Khubchandani, Kareem. *Ishtyle: Accenting Gay Indian Nightlife*. Ann Arbor: University of Michigan Press, 2020.

———. "Staging Transgender Solidarities at Bangalore's Queer Pride." *Transgender Studies Quarterly* 1, no. 4 (2014): 517–22.

———. "Voguing in Bangalore: Desire, Blackness, and Femininity in Globalized India." *Scholar & Feminist Online* 14, no. 3 (2018).

Khurana, Maya. "AIDS: From West to East?" *Nursing Journal of India* 77, no. 8 (1986): 207–13.

Kim-Puri, H. J. "Conceptualizing Gender-Sexuality-State-Nation: An Introduction." *Gender & Society* 19, no. 2 (2005): 137–59.

Klugman, Barbara. "The Politics of Contraception in South Africa." *Women's Studies International Forum* 13 (1990): 261–71.

Kole, Subir K. "Globalizing Queer? AIDS, Homophobia and the Politics of Sexual Identity in India." *Globalization and Health* 3, no. 8 (2007).

Kothari, Uma. "Authority and Expertise: The Professionalisation of International Development and the Ordering of Dissent." *Antipode* 37, no. 3 (2005): 425–46.

Kotiswaran, Prabha. *Dangerous Sex, Invisible Labor: Sex Work and the Law in India*. Princeton, NJ: Princeton University Press, 2011.

———."Has the Dial Moved on Indian Sex Work Debates?" *Economic & Political Weekly* 54, no. 22 (2019): 10–12.

———,ed. *Sex Work*. New Delhi: Women Unlimited, 2011.

Krause, Monika. *The Good Project: Humanitarian Relief NGOs and the Fragmentation of Reason*. Chicago: University of Chicago Press, 2014.

———."How Fields Vary." *British Journal of Sociology*, 2017.

Kreiss, Joan K., Davy Koech, Francis A. Plummer, King K. Holmes, Marilyn Lightfoote, Peter Piot, Allan R. Ronald, Josiah O. Ndinya-Achola, Lourdes J. D'Costa, and Pacita Roberts. "AIDS Virus Infection in Nairobi Prostitutes." *New England Journal of Medicine* 314, no. 7 (1986): 414–18.

KSAPS. *Annual Action Plan 2012–2013*. Bangalore: Karnataka State AIDS Prevention Society, 2011.

Kudva, Neema. "Strong States, Strong NGOs." In *Social Movements in India: Poverty, Power, and Politics*, by Raka Ray and Mary Katzenstein, 233–66. New York: Rowman & Littlefield, 2005.

———."Uneasy Relations," 2005.

Lakkimsetti, Chaitanya. "'HIV Is Our Friend': Prostitution, Power and State in Postcolonial India." *Signs: Journal of Women in Culture and Society* 40, no. 1 (2014): 201–26.

———.*Legalizing Sex: Sexual Minorities, AIDS, and Citizenship in India*. New York: New York University Press, 2020.

Lal, S., and T. E. Mertens. "HIV and AIDS." *Indian Journal of Public Health* 39, no. 3 (1995): 77–78.

Lancet. "India: Prostitutes and the Spread of AIDS." *Lancet* 335, no. 8701 (1990): 1332.

———."What Has the Gates Foundation Done for Global Health?" *Lancet* 373, no. 9675 (2009): 1577.

Latour, Bruno. *Science in Action: How to Follow Engineers and Scientists through Society*. Cambridge: Harvard University Press, 1987.

Lawyer's Collective. "Statement from the National Consultation on Sex Work, HIV and the Law," 2007.

Lee, Ching Kwan. "Raw Encounters: Chinese Managers, African Workers and the Politics of Casualization in Africa's Chinese Enclaves." *China Quarterly* 199 (2009): 647–66.

Legg, Stephen. *Prostitution and the Ends of Empire: Scale, Governmentalities, and Interwar India*. Durham, NC: Duke University Press, 2014.

Leigh, Carol. "Inventing Sex Work," in *Whores and Other Feminists*, ed. Jill Nagle. (New York: Routledge, 1997), 223–31.

Levine, Philippa. "'A Multitude of Unchaste Women:' Prostitution in the British Empire." *Journal of Women's History* 15, no. 4 (2004): 159–63.

———. *Prostitution, Race, and Politics: Policing Venereal Disease in the British Empire*. New York: Routledge, 2003.

———. "Rereading the 1890s: Venereal Disease as 'Constitutional Crisis' in Britain and British India." *Journal of Asian Studies* 55, no. 3 (1996): 585–612.

———. "Venereal Disease, Prostitution, and the Politics of Empire: The Case of British India." *Journal of the History of Sexuality* 4, no. 4 (1994): 579–602.

Lorway, Robert. "Making Global Health Knowledge: Documents, Standards, and Evidentiary Sovereignty in HIV Interventions in South India." *Critical Public Health* 27, no. 2 (2017): 1–16.

Lorway, Robert, and Shamshad Khan. "Reassembling Epidemiology: Mapping, Monitoring and Making-Up People in the Context of HIV Prevention in India." *Social Science & Medicine* 112 (2014): 51–62.

Lurie, Mark N., Brian G. Williams, Khangelani Zuma, David Mkaya-Mwamburi, Geoff P. Garnett, Adriaan W. Sturm, Michael D. Sweat, Joel Gittelsohn, and Salim S. Abdool Karim. "The Impact of Migration on HIV-1 Transmission in South Africa: A Study of Migrant and Nonmigrant Men and Their Partners." *Sexually Transmitted Diseases* 30, no. 2 (2003): 149–56.

Mahajan, Manjari. "Designing Epidemics: Models, Policy-Making, and Global Foreknowledge in India's AIDS Epidemic." *Science and Public Policy* 35, no. 8 (2008): 585–596.

———. "Philanthropy and the Nation-State in Global Health: The Gates Foundation in India." *Global Public Health* 13, no. 10 (2018): 1357–68.

Mahmood, Saba. *Politics of Piety*. Princeton, NJ: Princeton University Press, 2004.

Mai, Nicola. *Mobile Orientations: An Intimate Autoethnography of Migration, Sex Work, and Humanitarian Borders*. Chicago: University of Chicago Press, 2018.

Malik, S. R. K. "The Way Fatal AIDS Disease Spreads." *Times of India*, November 16, 1985.

Mandhani, Apoorva. "Anti-Trafficking Bill 2018—Do Not Equate Victims of Sex Trafficking with Voluntary Adult Sex Workers: MP Shashi Tharoor, Activists Appeal to WCD." *LiveLaw*. July 10, 2018.

Mangla, B. "India: Disquiet about AIDS Control." *Lancet* 340, no. 8834–8835 (1992): 1533–34.

Marks, Shula. "An Epidemic Waiting to Happen? The Spread of HIV/AIDS in South Africa in Social and Historical Perspective." *African Studies* 61, no. 1 (2002): 13–26.

Massey, Doreen. *Space, Place, and Gender.* Minneapolis: University of Minnesota Press, 1994.

Mathur, Nayanika. *Paper Tiger.* New York: Cambridge University Press, 2016.

McCann, Gerard. "Ties That Bind or Binds That Tie? India's African Engagements and the Political Economy of Kenya." *Review of African Political Economy* 37, no. 126 (2010): 465–82.

McCormick, Dorothy. "China & India as Africa's New Donors: The Impact of Aid on Development." *Review of African Political Economy* 35, no. 115 (2008): 73–92.

McDonnell, Erin Metz. "Patchwork Leviathan: How Pockets of Bureaucratic Governance Flourish within Institutionally Diverse Developing States." *American Sociological Review* 82, no. 3 (2017): 476–510.

McDonnell, Terence E. *Best Laid Plans: Cultural Entropy and the Unraveling of AIDS Media Campaigns.* Chicago: University of Chicago Press, 2016.

McGoey, Linsey. No Such Thing as a Free Gift: The Gates Foundation and the Price of Philanthropy. London: Verso, 2015.

McNeil, Donald, Jr. "India, Said to Play Down AIDS, Has Many Fewer With Virus Than Thought, Study Finds." *New York Times*, June 8, 2007.

Mehra, D. S. "Problems of AIDS in Developing Countries." *Journal of the Indian Medical Association* 93, no. 3 (1995): 115.

Mehta, J. "400 Million Condoms Diverted to Toy Manufacturers in India." *Journal of the International Association of Physicians in AIDS Care* 1, no. 1 (1995): 27.

Menon, Nivedita. "Sexuality, Caste, Governmentality: Contests over 'Gender' in India." *Feminist Review* 91, no. 1 (2009): 94–112.

Merry, Sally Engle. *The Seductions of Quantification: Measuring Human Rights, Gender Violence, and Sex Trafficking.* Chicago: University of Chicago Press, 2016.

Mgbako, Chi. *To Live Freely in This World: Sex Worker Activism in Africa.* New York: New York University Press, 2016.

Misra, Kavita. "Politico-Moral Transactions in Indian AIDS Service: Confidentiality, Rights and New Modalities of Governance." *Anthropological Quarterly* 79, no. 1 (2006): 33–74.

Mitchell, Timothy. "Society, Economy, and the State Effect." In *State/Culture: State-Formation after the Cultural Turn,* edited by George Steinmetz, 76–97. Ithaca, NY: Cornell University Press, 1999.

Mitra, Durba. *Indian Sex Life.* Princeton, NJ: Princeton University Press, 2020.

Mohan, Giles, and Kristiann Stokke. "Participatory Development and Empowerment: The Dangers of Localism." *Third World Quarterly* 21, no. 2 (2000): 247–68.

Mohan, Sadhna. "The AIDS Scare in India Could Be Aid-Induced." *Times of India*, September 19, 1996.

Mohan, Sunil. *Towards Gender Inclusivity: A Study of Contemporary Concerns around Gender.* Bangalore: Alternative Law Forum and LesBiT, 2013.

Mohanty, Chandra Talpade. "Under Western Eyes: Feminist Scholarship and Colonial Discourses." *Feminist Review* 30 (1988): 61–88.

———. "'Under Western Eyes' Revisited: Feminist Solidarity through Anticapitalist Struggles." *Signs: Journal of Women in Culture and Society* 28, no. 2 (2002): 499–535.

Mojola, Sanyu A. *Love, Money, and HIV: Becoming a Modern African Woman in the Age of AIDS.* Berkeley: University of California Press, 2014.

Morfit, N. S. "'AIDS Is Money': How Donor Preferences Reconfigure Local Realities." *World Development* 39, no. 1 (2011): 64–76.

Morgan, Kimberly J., and Ann Shola Orloff. *The Many Hands of the State: Theorizing Political Authority and Social Control.* New York: Cambridge University Press, 2017.

Moses, Stephen, Banadakoppa M. Ramesh, Nico JD Nagelkerke, Ajay Khera, Shajy Isac, Parinita Bhattacharjee, Vandana Gurnani, Reynold Washington, Kudur H. Prakash, and Banandur S. Pradeep. "Impact of an Intensive HIV Prevention Programme for Female Sex Workers on HIV Prevalence among Antenatal Clinic Attenders in Karnataka State, South India: An Ecological Analysis." *AIDS* 22 (2008): S101–8.

Mount, Liz. "'I Am Not a Hijra': Class, Respectability, and the Emergence of the 'New' Transgender Woman in India." *Gender & Society* 34, no. 4 (2020): 620–47.

Mudur, G.S. "Prevention Proof in HIV Study: 100,000 Cases Averted by Gates Foundation." *Telegraph*, December 10, 2011.

Murmu, L. R. "AIDS: Donors Dictate Third-World Strategy." *Lancet* 341, no. 8847 (1993): 764.

Murthy, Laxmi, and Meena Saraswathi Seshu. *The Business of Sex.* New Delhi: Zubaan, 2014.

NACC. "Kenya AIDS Strategic Framework 2014/2015–2018/2019." Nairobi: Ministry of Health, 2015.

———. *Kenya National AIDS Strategic Plan 2009/10–2012/13: Delivering on Universal Access to Services.* Nairobi: National AIDS Control Council, 2009.

———. *Kenya National AIDS Strategic Plan 2009/10-2012/13: Supporting*

Documents for the Strategic Plan. Nairobi: National AIDS Control Council, 2009.

———. *The Kenya National HIV/AIDS Strategic Plan 2000–2005.* Nairobi: National AIDS Control Council, 2000.

———. *Kenya National HIV/AIDS Strategic Plan 2005/6–2009/10: A Call to Action.* Nairobi: National AIDS Control Council, 2005.

NACO. "Funds and Expenditure." Accessed 2014. http://naco.gov.in/about-us/funds-and-expenditures-o.

———. *NACP III: To Halt and Reverse the HIV Epidemic in India.* New Delhi: National AIDS Control Organisation, Department of AIDS Control, Ministry of Health and Family Welfare, 2006.

———. *National AIDS Control Policy.* New Delhi: National AIDS Control Organisation, Department of AIDS Control, Ministry of Health and Family Welfare, 1999.

———. "National AIDS Control Programme IV." Accessed 2019. http://www.naco.gov.in/nacp.

———. National AIDS Control Programme Phase-IV (2012–2017): Strategy Document. New Delhi: Department of AIDS Control, Ministry of Health and Family Welfare. http://naco.gov.in/sites/default/files/Strategy_Document_NACP%20IV.pdf.

———. *National AIDS Control Programme Phase IV: Strategic Approach for Targeted Intervention among Female Sex Workers.* New Delhi: National AIDS Control Organisation, Department of AIDS Control, Ministry of Health and Family Welfare, 2011.

———. *National AIDS Control Programme: Response to the HIV Epidemic in India.* New Delhi: National AIDS Control Organisation, Department of AIDS Control, Ministry of Health and Family Welfare, 2010.

———. *National AIDS Prevention and Control Policy.* New Delhi: National AIDS Control Organisation, Ministry of Health and Family Welfare, 2003.

———. "NGO/CBO Operational Guidelines—Selection." New Delhi: Ministry of Health and Family Welfare, 2007.

———. *Targeted Interventions under NACP III Operational Guidelines. Volume 1: Core High Risk Groups.* New Delhi: National AIDS Control Organisation, Department of AIDS Control, Ministry of Health and Family Welfare, 2007.

NACO and ICMR. "India HIV Estimations 2017 Technical Report." New Delhi: National AIDS Control Organisation, Ministry of Health and Family Welfare, 2018.

Naidu, Sanusha. "India's Growing African Strategy." *Review of African Political Economy* 35, no. 115 (2008): 116–28.

Nair, Janaki. "The Devadasi, Dharma and the State." *Economic and Political Weekly* 29, no. 50 (1994): 3157–67.

———. *Mysore Modern: Rethinking the Region under Princely Rule.* Minneapolis: University of Minnesota Press, 2011.

———. *The Promise of the Metropolis: Bangalore's Twentieth Century.* New York: Oxford University Press, 2005.

Narlikar, Amrita. "India's Rise to Power: Where Does East Africa Fit In?" *Review of African Political Economy* 37, no. 126 (2010): 451–64.

Narrain, Arvind. "The Articulation of Rights around Sexuality and Health: Subaltern Queer Cultures in India in the Era of Hindutva." *Health and Human Rights* 7, no. 2 (2004): 142–64.

Narrain, Arvind, and Vinay Chandra. *Nothing to Fix: Medicalisation of Sexual Orientation and Gender Identity.* New Delhi: SAGE Publications, 2015.

NASCOP. *HIV/AIDS and Sexually Transmitted Infection in Kenya: Behavioural Surveillance Survey 2002 Summary Report.* Nairobi: National AIDS/STI Control Program, Ministry of Health, 2005.

———. *Kenya AIDS Indicator Survey 2007.* Nairobi: National AIDS and STI Control Programme, 2009.

———. *National Guidelines for HIV/STI Programs for Sex Workers.* Nairobi: Ministry of Public Health and Sanitation, 2010.

Nataraj, Shyamala. "Indian Prostitutes Highlight AIDS Dilemma." *Development Forum* 18, no. 1 (1990): 16.

National Intelligence Council. "The Next Wave of HIV/AIDS: Nigeria, Ethiopia, Russia, India, and China." Washington, DC: National Intelligence Officer for Economics and Global Issues, 2002.

National Network of Sex Workers. "Clarification Sought from the Justice Verma Committee," February 6, 2013. http://nnswindia.org/upload/News/Press-Release/JVC-Section-370IPC-Clarification.pdf.

———. "#SexWorkersAdviseHarvardYale." *National Network of Sex Workers India* (blog), July 13, 2020. https://medium.com/@nnswdelhi/sexworkersadviseharvardyale-827861f37968.

Naz Foundation. "Story of Naz." Accessed 2014. https://nazindia.org/.

New York Times. "71 AIDS Cases Recorded in India." February 15, 1987.

———. "Africa Students Protest AIDS Testing in India." *Metropolitan News*, 1987.

Ng, Marie, Emmanuela Gakidou, Alison Levin-Rector, Ajay Khera, Christopher J. L. Murray, and Lalit Dandona. "Assessment of Population-Level Effect of Avahan, an HIV-Prevention Initiative in India." *Lancet* 378, no. 9803 (2011): 1643–52.

Nguyen, Vinh-Kim. "Government-by-Exception: Enrolment and Experimentality in Mass HIV Treatment Programmes in Africa." *Social Theory & Health* 7, no. 3 (2009): 196–217.

———. *The Republic of Therapy: Triage and Sovereignty in West Africa's Time of AIDS*. Durham, NC: Duke University Press, 2010.

O'Connell, Gráinne. "Introduction: Framing 'Post-AIDS' and Global Health Discourses in 2015 and Beyond." *Journal of Medical Humanities* 41, no. 2 (2020): 89–94.

Oldenburg, Veena Talwar. "Lifestyle as Resistance: The Case of the Courtesans of Lucknow, India." *Feminist Studies* 16, no. 2 (1990): 259–87.

O'Manique, Colleen. "Global Neoliberalism and AIDS Policy: International Responses to Sub-Saharan Africa's Pandemic." *Studies in Political Economy* 73 (2004): 47–68.

Padabidri, M. K. "AIDS Threat." *Times of India*, July 10, 1986.

Padilla, Mark. *Caribbean Pleasure Industry: Tourism, Sexuality, and AIDS in the Dominican Republic*. Chicago: University of Chicago Press, 2008.

Padki, K. "Controlling AIDS in India." *BMJ* 308, no. 6941 (1994): 1436–37.

Pai, Aarthi. "Of a Pledge and a People." *The Hindu*, July 2, 2013.

Pais, Prem. "HIV and India: Looking into the Abyss." *Tropical Medicine and International Health* 1, no. 3 (1996): 295–304.

Pandit, Maya. "Gendered Subaltern Sexuality and the State." *Economic and Political Weekly* 48, no. 32 (2013): 33–38.

Parakal, Anthony. "AIDS Threat." *Times of India*, July 10, 1986.

Paschel, Tianna. "Disaggregating the Racial State: Activists, Diplomats, and the Partial Shift toward Racial Equality in Brazil." In *The Many Hands of the State: Theorizing Political Authority and Social Control*, edited by Kimberly J. Morgan and Ann Shola Orloff, 203–25. New York: Cambridge University Press, 2017.

Paschel, Tianna S. *Becoming Black Political Subjects: Movements and Ethno-Racial Rights in Colombia and Brazil*. Princeton, NJ: Princeton University Press, 2016.

Patil, Vrushali. "From Patriarchy to Intersectionality: A Transnational Feminist Assessment of How Far We've Really Come." *Signs: Journal of Women in Culture and Society* 38, no. 4 (2013): 847–67.

———. "The Heterosexual Matrix as Imperial Effect." *Sociological Theory* 36, no. 1 (2018): 1–26.

Patton, Cindy. "Inventing 'African AIDS.'" *New Formations*, no. 10 (1990): 25–39.

———. *Inventing AIDS*. New York: Routledge, 1991.

Payana. "Welcome to Payana." *Accessed 2020.* https://payanablr.in/.

Peck, Jamie, and Adam Tickell. "Neoliberalizing Space." *Antipode* 34, no. 3 (2002): 380–404.

Peck, Jamie, and Nik Theodore. "Follow the Policy: A Distended Case Approach." *Environment and Planning A* 44, no. 1 (2012): 21.

———. "Mobilizing Policy: Models, Methods, and Mutations." *Geoforum* 41, no. 2 (2010): 169–74.

———. "Recombinant Workfare, across the Americas: Transnationalizing 'Fast' Social Policy." *Geoforum* 41, no. 2 (2010): 195–208.

Peterson, V. Spike. "Political Identities/Nationalism as Heterosexism." *International Feminist Journal of Politics* 1, no. 1 (1999): 34–65.

Petryna, Adriana. "Experimentality: On the Global Mobility and Regulation of Human Subjects Research." *PoLAR: Political and Legal Anthropology Review* 30, no. 2 (2007): 288–304.

PFI, KSAPS, ICHAP, and PRB. *HIV/AIDS in Karnataka: Situation and Response.* Bangalore: Karnataka State AIDS Prevention Society, 2004.

Phadke, Shilpa, Sameera Khan, and Shilpa Ranade. *Why Loiter?: Women and Risk on Mumbai Streets.* New Delhi: Penguin Books India, 2011.

Pisani, Elizabeth, Geoff P. Garnett, Nicholas C. Grassly, Tim Brown, John Stover, Catherine Hankins, Neff Walker, and Peter D. Ghys. "Back to Basics in HIV Prevention: Focus on Exposure." *BMJ* 326, no. 7403 (2003): 1384–87.

Point of View. *Of Veshyas, Vamps, Whores, and Women.* Sangli: SANGRAM, 1998.

Prasada Rao, J. V. R. "Avahan: The Transition to a Publicly Funded Programme as a Next Stage." *Sexually Transmitted Infections* 86, no. 1 (2010): i7–8.

Priya, Ritu. "AIDS, Public Health, and the Panic Reaction (Part I)." *National Medical Journal of India* 7, no. 5 (1994): 235–40.

Puar, Jasbir K. *Terrorist Assemblages: Homonationalism in Queer Times.* Durham, NC: Duke University Press, 2018.

PUCL-K. *Human Rights Violations against the Transgender Community: A Study of Kothi and Hijra Sex Workers in Bangalore, Karnataka.* Bangalore: Peoples' Union for Civil Liberties, Karnataka, 2003.

———. *Policing Morality in Channapatna.* Bangalore: People's Union for Civil Liberties, Karnataka, 2007.

Puri, Jyoti. *Sexual States: Governance and the Struggle over the Antisodomy Law in India.* Durham, NC: Duke University Press, 2016.

Radhakrishnan, Smitha. *Appropriately Indian: Gender and Culture in a New Transnational Class.* Durham, NC: Duke University Press, 2011.

———. "Examining the 'Global' Indian Middle Class: Gender and Culture in the Silicon Valley/Bangalore Circuit." *Journal of Intercultural Studies* 29, no. 1 (2008): 7–20.

———. "'Time to Show Our True Colors': The Gendered Politics of 'Indianness' in Post-Apartheid South Africa." *Gender & Society* 19, no. 2 (2005): 262–81.

Rai, Shirin. "Gendering Global Governance." *International Feminist Journal of Politics* 6, no. 4 (2004): 579–601.

———. "Women and the State in the Third World." In *Women and Politics in the Third World*, edited by Haleh Afshar, 26–40. New York: Routledge, 1996.

Rajan, Rajeswari Sunder. *The Scandal of the State: Women, Law, and Citizenship in Postcolonial India*. Durham, NC: Duke University Press, 2003.

Ramberg, Lucinda. *Given to the Goddess: South Indian Devadasis and the Sexuality of Religion*. Durham, NC: Duke University Press, 2014.

———. "Magical Hair as Dirt: Ecstatic Bodies and Postcolonial Reform in South India." *Culture, Medicine, and Psychiatry* 33, no. 4 (2009): 501.

———. "When the Devi Is Your Husband: Sacred Marriage and Sexual Economy in South India." *Feminist Studies* 37, no. 1 (Spring 2011): 28–60, 223.

Rao, Sujatha. "How the LGBTQ Fight in India Went from Being a Health Issue to Civil Rights." *The Wire*, July 27, 2018.

Rau, Bill. *The Avahan-India AIDS Initiative: Promising Approaches to Combination HIV Prevention Programming in Concentrated Epidemics*. Arlington, VA: USAID and AIDSTAR-One, 2011.

Ray, Raka. *Fields of Protest: Women's Movements in India*. Minneapolis: University of Minnesota Press, 1999.

Ray, Raka, and Mary Fainsod Katzenstein. *Social Movements in India: Poverty, Power, and Politics*. New York: Rowman & Littlefield, 2005.

Reddy, Gayatri. *With Respect to Sex: Negotiating Hijra Identity in South India*. Chicago: University of Chicago Press, 2005.

Rege, Sharmila. "Dalit Women Talk Differently: A Critique of 'Difference' and towards a Dalit Feminist Standpoint Position." *Economic and Political Weekly* 33, no. 44 (1998): WS39–46.

Richardson, Diane. "Rethinking Sexual Citizenship." *Sociology* 51, no. 2 (2017): 208–24.

Rivers-Moore, Megan. "Waiting for the State: Sex Work and the Neoliberal Governance of Sexuality." *Social Politics* 21, no. 3 (2014): 403–29.

Robertson, James. "The Avahan Decade." *India HIV/AIDS Alliance* (blog), 2014. http://www.allianceindia.org/avahan-decade/.

Robins, Steven. "From 'Rights' to 'Ritual': AIDS Activism in South Africa." *American Anthropologist* 108, no. 2 (2006): 312–23.

Rose, Nikolas. "Governing by Numbers: Figuring out Democracy." *Accounting, Organizations and Society* 16, no. 7 (1991): 673–92.

Rottenburg, Richard. "Social and Public Experiments and New Figurations of Science and Politics in Postcolonial Africa." *Postcolonial Studies* 12, no. 4 (2009): 423–40.

Roy, Shubhajit. "India to its Missions: Don't Ask for HIV Tests of Visa Applicants." The Indian Express, November 27, 2010.

Roy, Srila. *New South Asian Feminisms: Paradoxes and Possibilities.* New Delhi: Aakar Books, 2017.

Roychowdhury, Poulami. *Capable Women, Incapable States.* New York: Oxford University Press, 2020.

———. "'The Delhi Gang Rape': The Making of International Causes." *Feminist Studies* 39, no. 1 (2013): 282–92.

RoyChowdhury, Supriya. "Bringing Class Back In: Informality in Bangalore." *Socialist Register* 51, no. 51 (2014).

Rubin, Gayle. "Thinking Sex: Notes for a Radical Theory of the Politics of Sexuality." In *Culture, Society and Sexuality: A Reader,* 143–79. New York: Taylor & Francis, 1997.

Sachan, Dinsa. "India's AIDS Department Merger Angers Activists." *Lancet* 384, no. 9946 (September 6, 2014): 842.

Sahni, Rohini, and V. Kalyan Shankar. *The First Pan-India Survey of Sex Workers: A Summary of Preliminary Findings.* Sangli: Center for Advocacy on Stigma and Marginalisation, 2011.

Sangama. "About Us." Accessed 2020. http://sangama.org/aboutus.html.

Sangaramoorthy, Thurka. "Treating the Numbers: HIV/AIDS Surveillance, Subjectivity, and Risk." *Medical Anthropology* 31, no. 4 (2012): 292–309.

Sangaramoorthy, Thurka, and Adia Benton. "Enumeration, Identity, and Health." *Medical Anthropology* 31, no. 4 (2012): 287–91.

SANGRAM. "About Us." Accessed 2018. https://www.sangram.org/about-us.

———. "Collectives." Accessed 2018. https://www.sangram.org/collectives.

———. "Submissions to Panels, Treaty Bodies, Commissions, and Government." 2018.

Say, Lale, Doris Chou, Alison Gemmill, Özge Tunçalp, Ann-Beth Moller, Jane Daniels, A. Metin Gülmezoglu, et al. "Global Causes of Maternal Death: A WHO Systematic Analysis." *Lancet Global Health* 2, no. 6 (2014): e323–33.

Schulman, Sarah. *The Gentrification of the Mind: Witness to a Lost Imagination.* Berkeley: University of California Press, 2012.

Sen, Amartya, Bill Gates, and Melinda Gates. *AIDS Sutra: Untold Stories from India.* New York: Anchor, 2008.

Sen, Simanta. "West Bengal Guards against AIDS." *Times of India,* October 16, 1985.

Seshu, Meena. "Collective Courages." Nairobi, 2015.

Sgaier, Sema K., Aparajita Ramakrishnan, Neeraj Dhingra, Alkesh Wadhwani, Ashok Alexander, Sara Bennett, Aparajita Bhalla, et al. "How the Avahan

HIV Prevention Program Transitioned from the Gates Foundation to the Government of India." *Health Affairs* 32, no. 7 (2013): 1265–73.

Sgaier, Sema K., Mariam Claeson, Charles Gilks, Banadakoppa M. Ramesh, Peter D. Ghys, Alkesh Wadhwani, Aparajita Ramakrishnan, Annie Tangri, and K. Chandramouli. "Knowing Your HIV/AIDS Epidemic and Tailoring an Effective Response: How Did India Do It?" *Sexually Transmitted Infections* 88, no. 4 (2012): 240–49.

Shah, Svati. "Sex Workers' Rights and Women's Movements in India: A Very Brief Genealogy." In *New South Asian Feminisms: Paradoxes and Possibilities*, 27–43. New Delhi: Aakar Books, 2017.

Shahani, Nishant. "How to Survive the Whitewashing of AIDS: Global Pasts, Transnational Futures." *QED: A Journal in GLBTQ Worldmaking* 3, no. 1 (2016): 1–33.

Sharma, Aradhana. "Crossbreeding Institutions, Breeding Struggle: Women's Empowerment, Neoliberal Governmentality, and State (Re)Formation in India." *Cultural Anthropology* 21, no. 1 (2006): 60–95.

———. *Logics of Empowerment: Development, Gender, and Governance in Neoliberal India*. Minneapolis: University of Minnesota Press, 2008.

Sheth, Anisha. "Sex, Sex Workers, and the City: The Double Standards of Desire and Respectability in Bengaluru." *News Minute*, July 26, 2015.

Shreedhar, J. "Dallying with Death: The Impending Crisis in India." *AIDScaptions* 1, no. 3 (1994): 16–19.

Shukla, Anuprita, Paul Teedon, and Flora Cornish. "Empty Rituals? A Qualitative Study of Users' Experience of Monitoring & Evaluation Systems in HIV Interventions in Western India." *Social Science & Medicine* 168, (2016): 7–15.

SIAAP. "The SIAAP Story." Accessed August 26, 2019. http://siaapindia.org.

Siddiqi, Dina M. "Sexuality, Rights and Personhood: Tensions in a Transnational World." *BMC International Health and Human Rights* 11, no. S3 (2011): S5.

Sidibé, Michel, Peter Piot, and Mark Dybul. "AIDS Is Not Over." *Lancet* 380, no. 9859 (2012): 2058–60.

Simmons, Beth A., Frank Dobbin, and Geoffrey Garrett. "The Global Diffusion of Public Policies: Social Construction, Coercion, Competition or Learning?" *Annual Review of Sociology* 33 (2007): 449–72.

Sindhu, Arman. "Modi Doctrine and the Future of Indo-African Ties." *Geopolitical Monitor*, 2020.

Singer, Merrill. *Introduction to Syndemics: A Critical Systems Approach to Public and Community Health*. Hoboken, NJ: John Wiley & Sons, 2009.

Smith, Faith L. *Sex and the Citizen: Interrogating the Caribbean*. Charlottesville: University of Virginia Press, 2011.

Smith, Julia H., and Alan Whiteside. "The History of AIDS Exceptionalism." *Journal of the International AIDS Society* 13, no. 1 (2010): 47.

Songok, E. M., S. A. Oogo, C. W. Mutura, E. M. Muniu, E. C. Koimett, D. L. Libondo, P. M. Tukei, and D. K. Koech. "Passage to India: The HIV Blockade on Kenyan Students." *AIDS* 8, no. 1 (1994): 138.

Sontag, Susan. *AIDS and Its Metaphors.* New York: Farrar, Straus and Giroux, 1989.

Srinivas, Smriti. *Landscapes of Urban Memory: The Sacred and the Civic in India's High-Tech City.* New Delhi: Orient Blackswan, 2004.

Steinmetz, George. "The Colonial State as a Social Field: Ethnographic Capital and Native Policy in the German Overseas Empire before 1914." *American Sociological Review* 73, no. 4 (2008): 589–612.

———. "The Octopus and the Hekatonkheire: On Many-Armed States and Tentacular Empires." In *The Many Hands of the State: Theorizing Political Authority and Social Control,* edited by Kimberly J. Morgan and Ann Shola Orloff, 369–93. New York: Cambridge University Press, 2017.

Strang, David, and John W. Meyer. "Institutional Conditions for Diffusion." *Theory and Society* 22, no. 4 (1993): 487–511.

Surya. "The Failed Radical Possibilities of Queerness in India." *Raiot,* February 3, 2016. http://www.raiot.in/the-failed-radical-possibilities-of-queerness-in-india.

Swabhava. "About." Accessed 2019. swabhava.org.

Swasti. "Chapter 15: Swathi Jyoti Receives an Award for Best Urban Micro Enterprise." #15YearsOfImpact. Bangalore: Swasti, 2019. https://swasti.org/swathi-jyoti-receives-an-award-for-best-urban-micro-enterprise/#.

Swidler, Ann, and Susan Cotts Watkins. *A Fraught Embrace: The Romance and Reality of AIDS Altruism in Africa.* Princeton, NJ: Princeton University Press, 2017.

SWOP–Kenya. "Who We Are." Accessed 2014. www.swop-kenya.org/services.

Tambe, Ashwini. *Codes of Misconduct: Regulating Prostitution in Late Colonial Bombay.* Minneapolis: University of Minnesota Press, 2009.

———. "The Elusive Ingénue: A Transnational Feminist Analysis of European Prostitution in Colonial Bombay." *Gender & Society* 19, no. 2 (2005): 160–79.

Tanne, J. H. "AIDS Spreads Eastward." *BMJ* 302, no. 6792 (1991): 1557.

Thomas, Rachel. "Spotlight on Meena Seshu, SANGRAM: Sex Worker Rights in Rural India." *Open Society Foundations: Voices* (blog), 2006. www.opensocietyfoundations.org/voices/spotlight-meena-seshu-sangram-sex-worker-rights-rural-india.

Thompson, Laura, Parinita Bhattacharjee, John Anthony, Mrunal Shetye, Stephen

Moses, and James Blanchard. *A Systematic Approach to the Scale-Up of Targeted Interventions for HIV Prevention Among Urban Female Sex Workers.* Bangalore: KHPT, 2012.

Times of India. "AIDS and Dinosaurs." December 24, 1994.

———. "AIDS Centre for Madras Hospital." May 1, 1986.

———. "AIDS Vaccine Not a Breakthrough Yet." October 19, 1985.

———. "AIDS Will Spread to Heterosexuals: Around the World." May 12, 1985.

———. "Blood Transfusion Test for AIDS." May 4, 1985.

———. "Coming to the AIDS of Asia: The AIDS Epidemic, Cutting Its Deathly Swathe across the World, Has Moved from the Gay Communities of San Francisco and Entire Populations in Sub-Saharan Africa to Fill in Its Ominous Shadow Lines throughout the Asia-Pacific Region." November 15, 1992.

———. "Doctor Warns of AIDS Epidemic." August 1, 1985.

———. "Don't Import AIDS via Blood: Expert." December 1, 1985.

———. "Indian Sex Taboos Ward off AIDS." September 2, 1985.

———. "India's First AIDS Clinic at J.J." March 6, 1986.

———. "Russia Untouched by AIDS." October 8, 1985.

———. "Who's to Be Blamed for AIDS?" November 10, 1985.

———. "WHO to Set up AIDS Panel." November 4, 1985.

Treichler, Paula. "AIDS, Homophobia and Biomedical Discourse: An Epidemic of Signification." *Cultural Studies* 1, no. 3 (1987): 263–305.

UN. "Eradicating AIDS by 2030 Requires Balanced Prevention, Treatment, Care Policies, Speakers Say as High-Level General Assembly Meeting Continues." UN Press Release, June 9, 2016. www.un.org/press/en/2016/ga11788.doc.htm.

UNAIDS. "2.5 Million People Living with HIV in India." July 4, 2007. www.unaids.org/en/resources/presscentre/featurestories/2007/july/20070704indianewdata.

———. *2006 Report on the Global AIDS Epidemic.* Geneva: UNAIDS, 2006.

———. "Global HIV & AIDS Statistics: 2019 Fact Sheet." Geneva: UNAIDS, 2019.

———. "Global HIV & AIDS Statistics: 2020 Fact Sheet." Geneva: UNAIDS, 2020. www.unaids.org/en/resources/fact-sheet.

———. *Global Report: UNAIDS Report on the Global AIDS Epidemic 2010.* Geneva: UNAIDS, 2010.

———. "India Overview." Accessed 2018. www.unaids.org/en/regionscountries/countries/india.

———. "Miles to Go." Geneva: UNAIDS, 2018.

———. *Report on the Global AIDS Epidemic.* Geneva: UNAIDS, 2012.

———. *Report on the Global HIV/AIDS Epidemic 2008.* Geneva: UNAIDS, 2008.

———. "South Africa." Accessed 2020. www.unaids.org/en/regionscountries/countries/southafrica.

———. *UNAIDS Guidance Note on HIV and Sex Work*. Geneva: UNAIDS, 2007.

———. *UNAIDS Guidance Note on HIV and Sex Work*. Geneva: UNAIDS, 2012.

———. *UNAIDS Terminology Guidelines*. Geneva: UNAIDS, 2015.

UNAIDS and WHO. "AIDS Epidemic Update." Geneva: UNAIDS and WHO, 2004.

UNAIDS and WHO. *Report on the Global HIV/AIDS Epidemic June 1998*. Geneva: UNAIDS, 1998.

UNDP. "Eight Goals for 2015." Accessed 2020. www.in.undp.org/content/india/en/home/post-2015/mdgoverview.

Upadhya, Carol, and A. R. Vasavi. *In an Outpost of the Global Economy: Work and Workers in India's Information Technology Industry*. New Delhi: Routledge, 2012.

Vahed, Goolam. "The Making of Indianness: Indian Politics in South Africa during the 1930s and 1940s." *Journal of Natal and Zulu History* 17, no. 1 (1997): 1–36.

VAMP, SANGRAM, and Rights4Change. *Raided: How Anti-Trafficking Strategies Increase Sex Workers' Vulnerability to Exploitative Practices*. Sangli: SANGRAM, 2018.

Varam, D. "AIDS Situation Explosive in India, Say Doctors." *Aids Asia: Voice of the Asian Solidarity against AIDS* 3, no. 6 (1996): 9.

Verma, J. S., Leila Seth, and Gopal Subramanium. "Report of the Committee on Amendments to Criminal Law." New Delhi, January 23, 2013.

VHS, NACO, and KHPT. *GFATM Round 10 India HIV Country Proposal: Reduced Vulnerability of Most at Risk Populations to HIV by Enhancing the Quality and Scale of Interventions and Strengthening Community Systems*. Voluntary Health Services, National Aids Control Organization, and Karnataka Health Promotion Trust, 2010.

Vijaisri, Priyadarshini. "Contending Identities: Sacred Prostitution and Reform in Colonial South India." *South Asia: Journal of South Asian Studies* 28, no. 3 (2005): 387–411.

Vijayakumar, Gowri. "Collective Demands and Secret Codes: The Multiple Uses of 'Community' in 'Community Mobilization.'" *World Development* 104 (2018): 173–82.

———. "Is Sex Work Sex Or Is Sex Work Work? The Formation of the 'Sex Worker' in Bangalore." *Qualitative Sociology* 41, no. 3 (2018): 337–60.

———. "Sexual Laborers and Entrepreneurial Women: Articulating Collective

Identity in India's HIV/AIDS Response." *Social Problems* 67, no. 3 (2020): 507–26.

Vijayakumar, Gowri, Shubha Chacko, and Subadra Panchanadeswaran. "'As Human Beings and As Workers': Sex Worker Unionization in Karnataka, India." *Global Labour Journal* 6, no. 1 (2015).

Vimochana. "An Open Letter to the State Government from the Women of Karnataka." *UltraViolet* (blog), January 29, 2009. youngfeminists.wordpress.com/2009/01/29/an-open-letter-to-the-state-government-from-the-women-of-karnataka.

Virology Education. "Ishwar Gilada, MD, DDV, FCPS." Accessed August 28, 2019. www.virology-education.com/ishwar-gilada-md-ddv-fcps.

Viterna, Jocelyn. "Pulled, Pushed, and Persuaded: Explaining Women's Mobilization into the Salvadoran Guerrilla Army." *American Journal of Sociology* 112, no. 1 (2006): 1–45.

———. *Women in War: The Micro-Processes of Mobilization in El Salvador*. New York: Oxford University Press, 2013.

Watkins-Hayes, Celeste. "Intersectionality and the Sociology of HIV/AIDS: Past, Present, and Future Research Directions." *Annual Review of Sociology* 40, no. 1 (2014): 431–57.

———. *Remaking a Life*. Berkeley: University of California Press, 2018.

White, Luise. *The Comforts of Home: Prostitution in Colonial Nairobi*. Chicago: University of Chicago Press, 1990.

Whitehead, Judy. "Bodies Clean and Unclean: Prostitution, Sanitary Legislation, and Respectable Femininity in Colonial North India." *Gender & History* 7, no. 1 (1995): 41–63.

WHO. "Contributors." Accessed January 11, 2021. open.who.int/2020-21/contributors/contributor.

———. "Global Health Estimates 2016: Deaths by Cause, Age, Sex, by Country and by Region, 2000–2016." Geneva: World Health Organization, 2018.

———. "India Taken off WHO's List of Polio Endemic Countries." SEARO. February 25, 2012. origin.searo.who.int/immunization/topics/polio/polio_summit_india/en.

———. "India Three Years Polio-Free." SEARO, March 27, 2014. http://www.searo.who.int/mediacentre/features/2014/sea-polio/en.

———. *Preventing HIV among Sex Workers in Sub-Saharan Africa: A Literature Review*. Geneva: World Health Organization, 2011.

WHO, UNICEF, UNFPA, World Bank, and UNFPA. "Trends in Maternal Mortality: 1990–2015." Geneva: World Health Organization, 2015.

Wines, Michael. "Durban Journal; As AIDS Continues to Ravage, South Africa 'Recycles' Graves." *New York Times*, July 29, 2004.

Woods, Ngaire. "Whose Aid? Whose Influence? China, Emerging Donors and the Silent Revolution in Development Assistance." *International Affairs* 84, no. 6 (2008): 1205–21.

World Bank. "Implementation Completion and Results Report (IDA-32420) on a Credit in the Amount of SDR 140.82 Million to India for Second National HIV/AIDS Control Project." New Delhi: South Asia Human Development Sector, World Bank, 2006.

———. "World Bank Open Data." Accessed 2017. data.worldbank.org.

Wyrod, Robert. *AIDS and Masculinity in the African City: Privilege, Inequality, and Modern Manhood.* Berkeley: University of California Press, 2016.

Yengkhom, Sumati. "Sex Worker Invited to Mamata's Swearing-in Ceremony." *Times of India.* May 19, 2011.

Yuval-Davis, Nira. "Gender and Nation." In *Women, Ethnicity and Nationalism*, edited by Rick Wilford and Robert L. Miller, 23–35. New York: Routledge, 2004.

Index

ABVA. *See* AIDS Bhedbhav Virodhi
  Andolan
activism: after AIDS crisis, 157; AIDS-
  related, 46, 55, 160; civil society
  organizations in relation to, 61–62;
  in Kenya, 148–50; for kothis, xii,
  81; for sexual minorities, xii; for
  sex workers, xii, 76–83, 148–50,
  160; for transgender people, xii, 81,
  160. *See also* feminist scholarship/
  activism; politics
Africa: AIDS associated with, 26–27;
  Indian AIDS situation compared
  to that in, vii, 13, 19–20, 27–35,
  123–51; India's relationship with,
  136–37, 151
African Sex Workers' Alliance, 149
AIDS Bhedbhav Virodhi Andolan
  (ABVA, Movement Against
  AIDS-Related Discrimination),
  7, 44, 53

AIDS in India: African situations
  compared to, xii, 13, 19–20, 27–35,
  123–51; heterosexual vs. homosexual means of transmitting, 26–27,
  36; opinions on severity of, 4–5,
  18–19, 29–36, 118–19, 152–56, 191n75;
  other diseases compared to, 4, 18;
  prevalence of, vii, xv, 4, 11, 18–19,
  35, 138, 153
AIDS Prevention Bill, 44
AIDS response/HIV prevention in
  India: Africans as early target of,
  28–29; assessments of, 111, 113–14,
  153; categorization of high-risk
  groups in, 7, 99–102, 195n32;
  complexity of, 12; containment
  strategy of, 41–45; critiques of,
  2, 4, 7, 99; development of, xi; in
  early years, 26, 28, 36; effects and
  implications of, ix, xv, 2, 8–9,
  14, 17, 41, 52–54, 62–65, 86–109,

GLOBALIZATION
IN EVERYDAY LIFE

As global forces undeniably continue to change the politics and economies of the world, we need a more nuanced understanding of what these changes mean in our daily lives. Significant theories and studies have broadened and deepened our knowledge on globalization, yet we need to think about how these macro processes manifest on the ground and how they are maintained through daily actions.

Globalization in Everyday Life foregrounds ethnographic examination of daily life to address issues that will bring tangibility to previously abstract assertions about the global order. Moving beyond mere illustrations of global trends, books in this series underscore mutually constitutive processes of the local and global by finding unique and informative ways to bridge macro- and microanalyses. This series is a high-profile outlet for books that offer accessible readership, innovative approaches, instructive models, and analytic insights to our understanding of globalization.

Here, There, and Elsewhere: The Making of Immigrant Identities in a Globalized World
    Tahseen Shams   **2020**

Beauty Diplomacy: Embodying an Emerging Nation
    Oluwakemi M. Balogun   **2020**

CPSIA information can be obtained
at www.ICGtesting.com
Printed in the USA
JSHW021121190722
28277JS00001B/53